The Complete Vegetarian Recipe Book

The Best Collection to Discover New Recipes and Improve Your Lifestyle

America Best Recipes

Table of Contents

Breakfast

Quinoa Breakfast Muffins

Prep time: 05 min Cooking Time: 10 min Serve: 2

Ingredients

1 cup cooked quinoa

2 eggs

1/2 cup chopped fresh spinach leaves

1 /2 cup cherry tomatoes

1/2 cup sliced mushrooms

1/2 cup cubed zucchini

1 1/2 grated parmesan cheese

Salt and pepper to taste

Cooking spray

1 cup of water

Instructions

Spray 6 (6-ounce) ovenproof custard cups with non-stick cooking spray.

In a large bowl, whisk the eggs, salt and pepper, until just blended. Evenly divide the cooked quinoa, spinach, cherry tomatoes, mushrooms, cheese and zucchini among the custard cups. Pour the egg mixture over the veggies.

Pour 1 cup of water into the Instant Pot cooking pot and place a trivet in the bottom. Place 2 custard cups on the trivet and place a second trivet on top. Place the remaining 2 cups on it. Lock lid in place. Select High Pressure and 6 minutes cook time.

When the cook time ends, turn off the instant cooker. Let the pressure release naturally for 5 minutes and finish with a quick pressure release. When the valve drops, carefully open the lid and remove the cups.

Nutrition Facts

Calories 439, Total Fat 12.7g, Saturated Fat 4g ,Cholesterol 174mg, , Sodium 208mg, Total Carbohydrate 59g , Dietary Fiber 7.2g, , Total Sugars 2.3g, Protein 23.6g

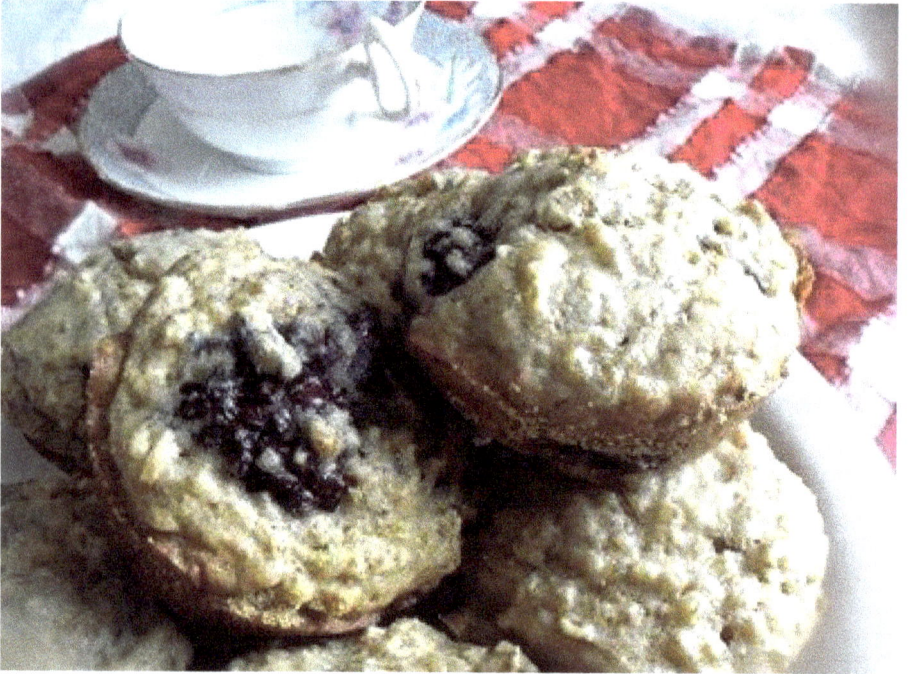

Almond Cherry Buckwheat

Prep time: 05 min Cooking Time: 10 min Serve: 2

Ingredients

1/8 teaspoon salt

1 cup buckwheat

1 cup pitted chopped cherries

1/3 cup toasted slivered almonds

2 tablespoon maple syrup (plus more to taste)

1 teaspoon almond extract

1 teaspoon chia seeds

Instructions

Pit and chop your cherries. Set a few aside for garnish.

Add all the ingredients to the Instant Pot, stirring the mixture together.

Lock lid on your Instant Pot.

Set the Instant Pot on Multigrain for 6 minutes, and let it cook and naturally release.

When the buckwheat has finished cooking.

Transfer buckwheat to bowls, top with extra chopped cherries, toasted slivered almonds, and chia seeds.

Nutrition Facts

Calories493, Total Fat 11.4g, Saturated Fat 1.3g, Cholesterol 0mg , Sodium 157mg, Total Carbohydrate 89g, Dietary Fiber 11.3g, Total Sugars 12.8g, Protein 15g

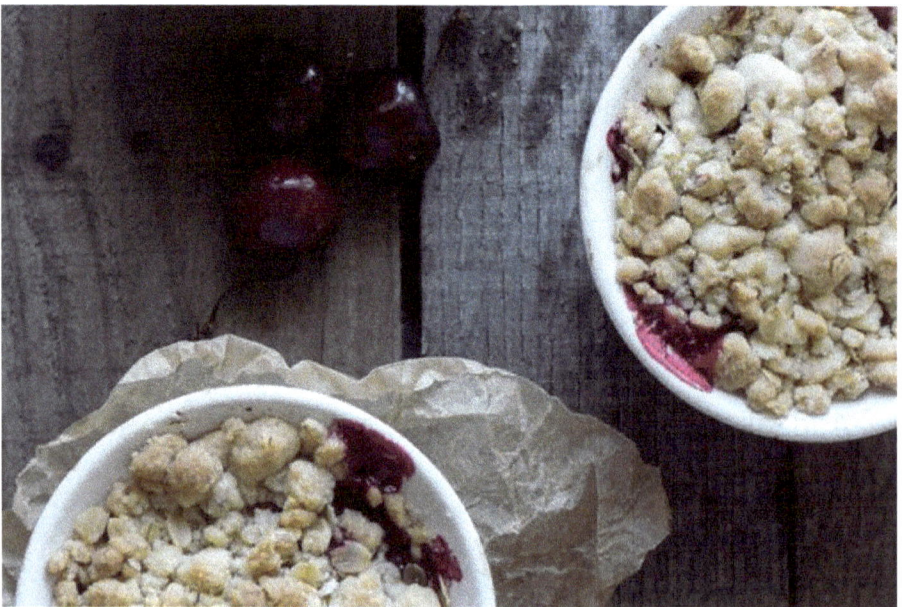

Eggs in Spinach and Tomato

Prep time: 10 min Cooking Time: 15 min Serve: 2

Ingredients

2 cups spinach

4 medium tomatoes

1 small onion

½ cup goat cheese

1 tablespoon coconut oil

½ cup parsley, fresh (chopped)

1 teaspoon red pepper flakes

Salt and pepper to taste

2 eggs

Instructions

Add all the ingredients except eggs to the Instant Pot, stirring the mixture together.

Crack the eggs and pour into the bowl.

Lock lid on your Instant Pot.

Set the Instant Pot on High Pressure for 10 minutes, and let it cook and naturally release.

Add another dash of salt and pepper to the top.

Enjoy.

Nutrition Facts

Calories 214, Total Fat 13.6g, Saturated Fat 8.4g, Cholesterol 167mg Sodium 133mg, Total Carbohydrate 15.8g, Dietary Fiber 5.1g, Total Sugars 8.7g, Protein 10.8g

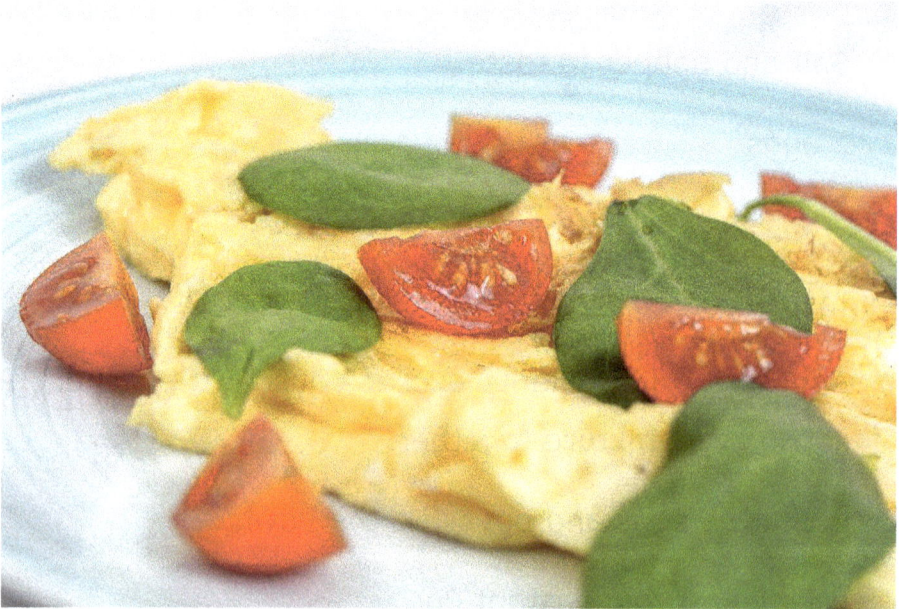

Kale Casserole

Prep time: 10 min Cooking Time: 20 min Serve: 2

Ingredients

2 eggs

1/8 teaspoon salt

1/16 teaspoon pepper

1 cup kale

¼ cup grated cheddar cheese

½ cup cauliflower

Cooking spray

1 cup of water

Instructions

In a bowl whisk together the eggs and add salt and pepper. Set aside.

Spray an oven safe dish with non-stick cooking spray. Add kale, cauliflower and cheddar cheese.

Pour the egg mixture over the top of everything.

Pour 1 cup of water in the bottom of your Instant Pot. Place a trivet in the bottom of the pot. Cover

your casserole pan loosely with foil. Use a foil sling or silicone sling to lower the pan into the Instant Pot, on top of the trivet.

Cover the Instant Pot and lock lid in place and turn the valve to Sealing. Press the Pressure Cooker button and set the cook time for 20 minutes at High Pressure. Let the pressure release naturally for 10 minutes and then move the valve to Venting.

Serve. Open the pot and carefully use the sling to remove the pan. Remove the foil. Cut the casserole

and serve.

Nutrition Facts

Calories143, Total Fat 9.1g, Saturated Fat 4.3g, Cholesterol 179mg , Sodium 319mg, Total Carbohydrate 5.4g, Dietary Fiber 1.2g , Total Sugars 1g, Protein 10.6g

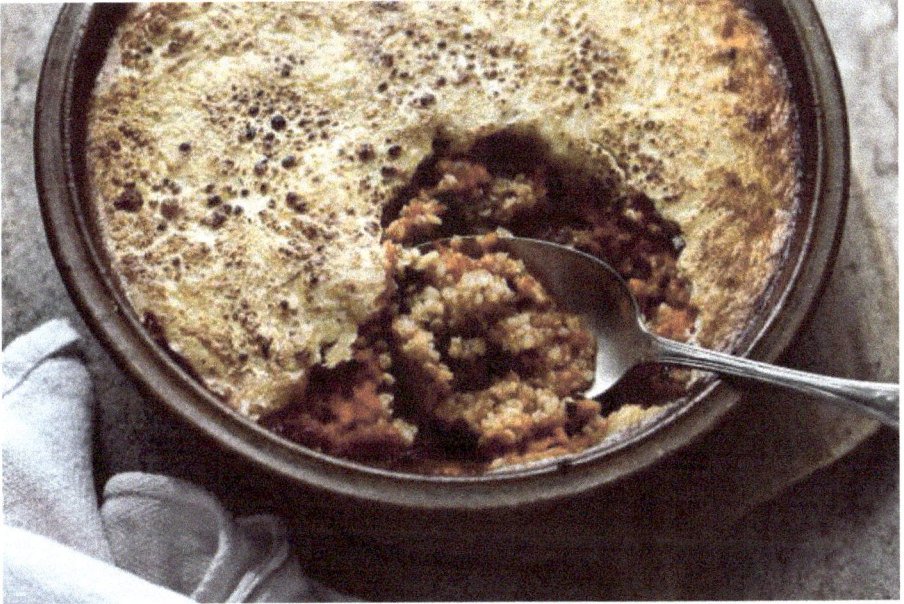

Pumpkin Buckwheat Porridge

Prep time: 05 min Cooking Time: 15 min Serve: 2

Ingredients

1 cup uncooked buckwheat

½ cup pureed pumpkin

1 teaspoon pumpkin pie spice

¼ teaspoon salt

¼ cup honey

¾ cup water

½ cup almond milk

½ tablespoon vanilla

2 cups water

Instructions

Place the buckwheat, pumpkin puree, pumpkin pie spice, salt, honey, water, almond milk and vanilla in the Instant Pot.

Lock lid. Set the pressure to "High". Move the valve to "Sealing‖ and cook for 15 minutes.

Once the timer has rung, allow the Instant Pot to sit (also known as naturally release pressure) for ten minutes. Once this is done, the timer will show.

Open the lid and stir to combine everything.

Serve warm.

Nutrition Facts

Calories 583, Total Fat 17.3g, Saturated Fat 13.4g, Cholesterol 0mg, Sodium 308mg, Total Carbohydrate 102.8g, Dietary Fiber 10.8g, Total Sugars 38.3g, Protein 13.3g

Breakfast Muffins

Preparation Time: 10 minutes Cooking time: 6 minutes Servings: 4

Ingredients

2 cups diced banana

½ cup coconut milk, unsweetened

¼ cup coconut oil, melted

1 cup frozen sliced strawberries

2 teaspoons maple syrup

1 tablespoon ground flaxseed

⅓ cup almond flour ½ cup dates

Directions:

Line muffin tins and set aside. Then add ground flax seeds, almond meal and dates into a food processor. Pulse the mixture until it becomes crumbly and then transfer to a bowl. Stir in maple syrup and then press a tablespoon of crust mixture into the bottom of the muffin gently, to make the crust.

Put semi-thawed strawberries in a food processor and pulse until smooth. Add in coconut and coconut milk slowly until you achieve a thick, sorbet consistency.

In a bowl, add in the strawberries and gently fold in the bananas. Then sub-divide the strawberry banana mixture over the top of the crust evenly.

Finally put the muffins in a freezer and let it freeze and solidify. Once frozen place in freezer bags and freeze. To serve, thaw for around 15 minutes and then serve

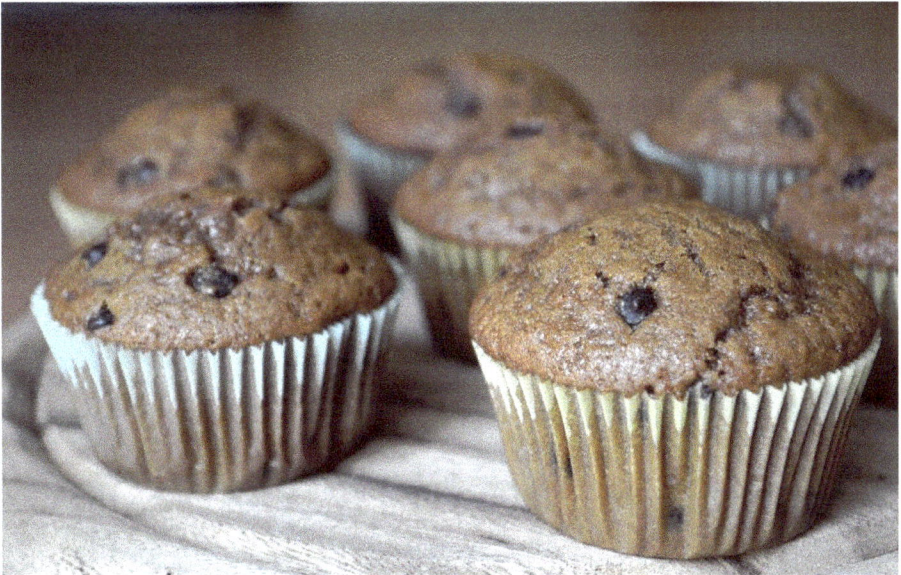

Bean Salsa Breakfast

Preparation Time: 10 minutes Cooking time: 6 minutes
Servings: 2

Ingredients

Olive oil ½ lemon 1 avocado

2 cloves of garlic

2 handfuls of spinach

1 handful of basil

6 cherry tomatoes

4 spring onions

1 can of haricot beans

Black pepper Himalayan salt

Directions:

Chop the onions and the garlic and then halve the cherry tomatoes. Let 50ml water to boil in a frying pan and then steam-fry the garlic for a few seconds. Throw in the spring onions, haricot beans and the cherry tomatoes and cook until soft. Now add in the spinach and basil and cook until wilted, season with the black pepper and Himalayan salt.

Meanwhile, halve the avocado. To serve, top the bean mixture with halved avocado and lemon. Alternatively, you can freeze the bean mixture for another day. When serving, top with an avocado and some lemon.

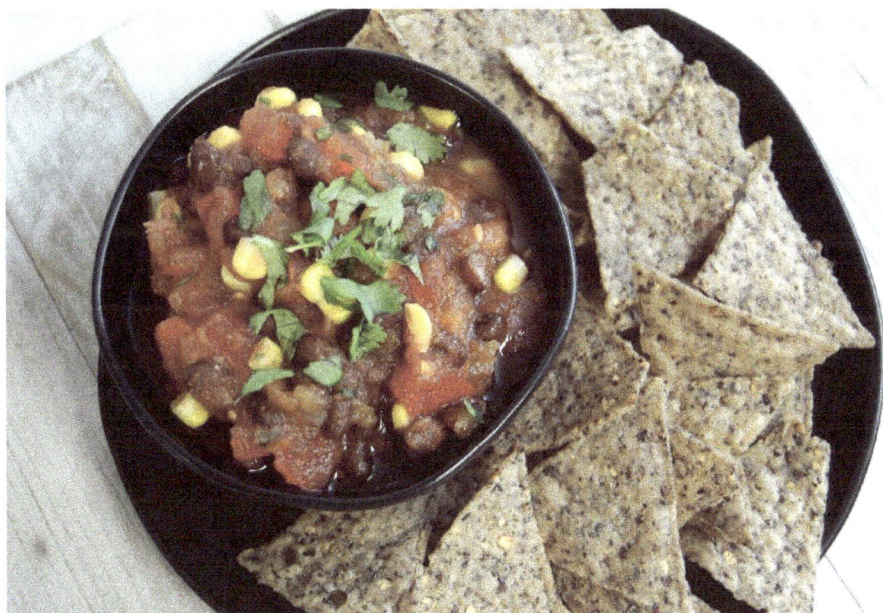

Gingerbread-Spiced Breakfast Smoothie

Preparation Time: 2 minutes Cooking Time: Servings: 2

Ingredients:

1 cup Coconut Milk

1 bag Tea ¼ tsp Cinnamon Powder

1/8 tsp Nutmeg Powder

1/8 tsp Powdered Cloves

1/3 cup Chia Seeds

2 tbsp Flax Seeds

Directions:

Put the teabag in a mug and pour in a cup of hot water. Allow to steep for a few minutes. Pour the tea into a blender together with the rest of the Ingredients. Process until smooth.

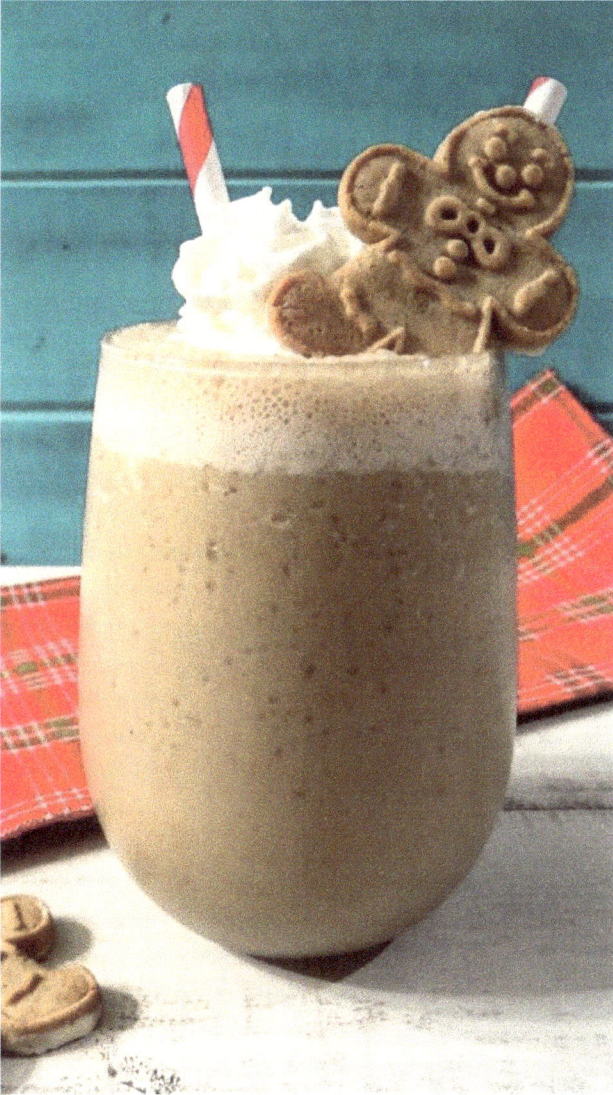

Maca Caramel Frap

Preparation time: 5 minutes Cooking time: 0 minute

Servings: 4

Ingredients:

1/2 of frozen banana, sliced

1/4 cup cashews, soaked for 4 hours

2 Medjool dates, pitted

1 teaspoon maca powder

1/8 teaspoon sea salt

1/2 teaspoon vanilla extract, unsweetened

1/4 cup almond milk, unsweetened

1/4 cup cold coffee, brewed

Directions:

Place all the ingredients in the order in a food processor or blender and then pulse for 2 to 3 minutes at high speed until smooth. Pour the smoothie into a glass and then serve.

Peach Crumble Shake

Preparation time: 5 minutes Cooking time: 0 minute Servings: 1

Ingredients:

1 tablespoon chia seeds

¼ cup rolled oats

2 peaches, pitted, sliced

¾ teaspoon ground cinnamon

1 Medjool date, pitted

½ teaspoon vanilla extract, unsweetened

2 tablespoons lemon juice ½ cup of water

1 tablespoon coconut butter 1 cup coconut milk, unsweetened

Directions:

Place all the ingredients in the order in a food processor or blender and then pulse for 2 to 3 minutes at high speed until smooth. Pour the smoothie into a glass and then serve.

Lunch
Braised Tofu with Mushrooms

Prep time: 10 min Cooking Time: 10 min Serve: 2)

Ingredients

1 cup tofu

2 tablespoons olive oil

½ cup pecans

1 cup mushrooms, stems removed

½ cup green peas

½ teaspoon soy sauce

1 cup water

Instructions

Slice tofu block into 3 long slabs lengthwise. Wrap each slab in paper towels and press to squeeze out excess water.

Select Sauté on the Instant Pot. When the Instant Pot is hot, add 1 tablespoon olive oil once the oil is hot, and add the tofu slabs to the pot. Fry for about 5 minutes on each side or until delicately browned. Set aside.

Remove tofu from the pot, and slice into cubes. Add the remaining teaspoon olive oil to the Instant Pot, and stir fry the pecans, mushrooms, and green

Peas. Mix water and soy sauce, and add to the pot along with the tofu.

Secure the lid on the pot. Close the pressure-release valve. Select Manual and set the pot at High Pressure for 5 minutes. At the end of the cooking time, allow the pot to sit undisturbed for 10 minutes, then release any remaining pressure.

Nutrition Facts

Calories 289, Total Fat 22g, Saturated Fat 3.4g, Cholesterol 0mg, Sodium 97mg, Total Carbohydrate

9.1g, Dietary Fiber 3.7g, Total Sugars 3.6g, Protein 13.8g

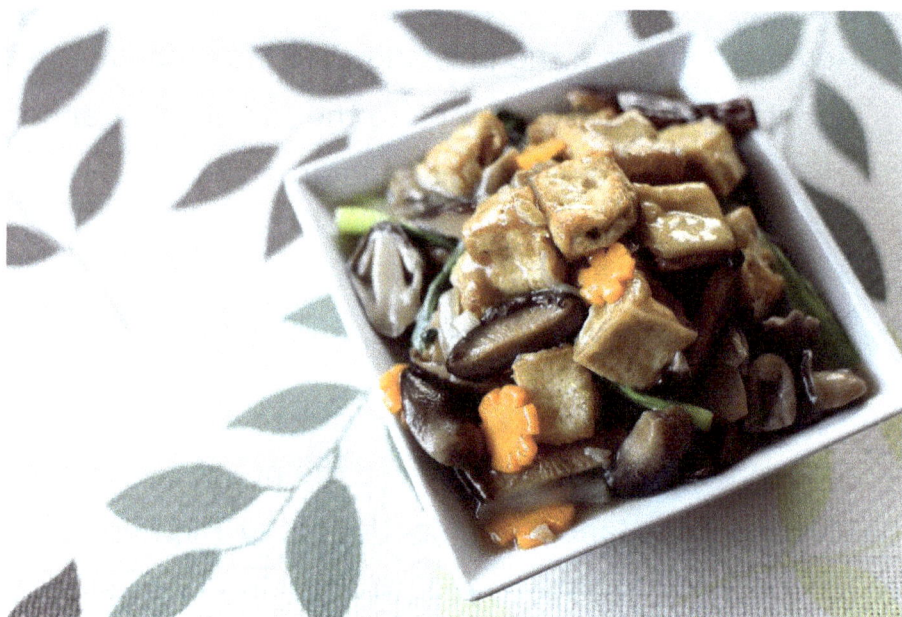

Tofu and Broccoli with Sesame Seed

Prep time: 5 min Cooking Time: 10 min Serve: 2

Ingredients

¼ cup soy sauce

1 cup vegetable broth

1 teaspoon honey

1 teaspoon garlic powder

½ teaspoon ginger powder

2 cups tofu

1 cup fresh bite-sized broccoli florets

2 teaspoons vegetable oil

1 tablespoon corn-starch

Sesame seeds for garnish

Instructions

Add soy sauce, vegetable broth, honey, garlic powder, and ginger powder to the pot and stir until well combined. Add tofu and toss to coat.

Secure the lid, making sure the vent is closed.

Using the display panel, select the Manual or Pressure Cook function. Use the + /- keys and program the Instant Pot for 5 minutes. When the time is up, quickly release the remaining pressure.

Remove ¼ cup of cooking liquid and mix with corn starch. Stir corn starch slurry, broccoli florets, and toasted sesame oil into the pot for 3-5 minutes until broccoli is tender and the sauce has thickened, returning to Sauté mode as needed. Garnish with sesame seeds.

Nutrition Facts

Calories 308, Total Fat 16g, Saturated Fat 3.3g, Cholesterol 0mg , Sodium 2225mg, Total Carbohydrate

14.4g, Dietary Fiber 3.9g , Total Sugars 6.4g, Protein 26.7g

Red Curry with Tofu and Lots of Vegetables

Prep time: 10 min Cooking Time: 20 min Serve: 2

Ingredients

1 cup tofu, cubed

1 tablespoon light soy sauce, or more to taste

1 cup coconut milk

½ tablespoon Thai red curry paste, or more to taste

1 cup broccoli florets

½ cup fresh mushrooms

1 green onion, cut lengthwise, washed, trimmed, and sliced thin

1 carrot, cut into matchsticks

1 lemon juice, or to taste

½ teaspoon honey

Instructions

Combine tofu and ½ tablespoon soy sauce in a small bowl and marinate for about 20 minutes. 2. Add coconut milk, Thai red curry paste, tofu, broccoli, mushrooms, green onion, and carrot mix well. Secure the lid, making sure the vent is closed.

Using the display panel, select the Manual or Pressure Cook function. Use the + /- keys and program

the Instant Pot for 5 minutes.

When the time is up, quickly release the remaining pressure. Season with soy sauce, lemon juice, and honey.

Nutrition Facts

Calories 536, Total Fat 40g, Saturated Fat 26.7g, Cholesterol 0mg , Sodium 3071mg, Total Carbohydrate 27.1g, Dietary Fiber 8.1g, Total Sugars 14.2g, Protein 17.4g

Mushrooms Tofu Stir-Fry

Prep time: 10 min Cooking Time: 15 min Serve: 2

Ingredients

1 cup tofu, cut into 1-inch cubes

½ tablespoon coconut oil

½ cup sliced fresh mushrooms

½ tablespoon chopped garlic

1 1/2 cups fresh kale

1 tablespoon soy sauce

1 tablespoon curry powder

½ teaspoon red pepper flakes

Instructions

Select Sauté on the Instant Pot. When the Instant Pot is hot, add coconut oil. Once the oil is hot, Add mushrooms and garlic; cook and stir until mushrooms are tender for 2-3 minutes. Add tofu, kale, soy sauce, and curry powder.

Secure the lid on the pot. Close the pressure-release valve. Select Manual and set the pot at High Pressure for 5 minutes. At the end of the cooking time, allow the pot to sit undisturbed for 10 minutes, then release any remaining. Sprinkle red pepper flakes over the mixture.

Nutrition Facts

Calories 160, Total Fat 9.3g, Saturated Fat 4.1g, Cholesterol 0mg, Sodium 481mg, Total Carbohydrate

6.6g, Dietary Fiber 2.9g, Total Sugars 1.4g, Protein 12.4g

Vegetarian Curry

Prep time: 15 min Cooking Time: 15 min Serve: 2

Ingredients

½ head cauliflower, chopped

1 cup green peas

2 potatoes, chopped

2 tomatoes, chopped

1 cup vegetable broth

½ teaspoon ground cumin

½ teaspoon curry powder

½ teaspoon turmeric powder

1/2 teaspoon chili powder

Instructions

Combine cauliflower, peas, potatoes, tomatoes, vegetable broth, ground cumin, curry powder, turmeric powder, and chili powder in an Instant Pot.

Secure the lid on the pot. Close the pressure-release valve. Select Manual and set the pot at High Pressure for 5 minutes. At the end of the cooking time, allow the pot to sit undisturbed for 10 minutes, then release any remaining.

Nutrition Facts

Calories 271, Total Fat 1.9g, Saturated Fat 0.4g, Cholesterol 0mg, Sodium 432mg, Total Carbohydrate

53.9g, Dietary Fiber 12.5g, Total Sugars 11.8g, Protein 12.6g

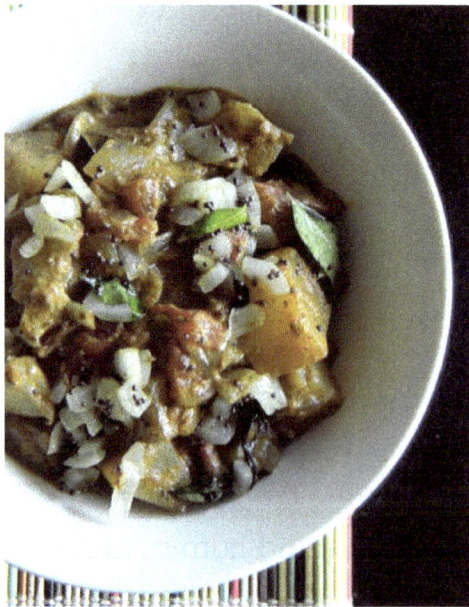

Zucchini and Eggplant Rice

Prep time: 10 min Cooking Time: 25 min serve: 2

Ingredients

2 tablespoons coconut oil

1 tablespoon almonds

¼ cup onion, sliced

1 green chili, chopped (or to taste)

½ tablespoon ginger garlic paste

1 tomato, chopped

½ cup eggplant, cubed

½ cup zucchini, cubed

1 cup basmati rice

2 cups water

1 teaspoon cumin seeds

1 tablespoon coriander powder

1 teaspoon Garam masala

salt to taste

Red chili powder to taste

Instructions

Press Sauté mode on High Pressure and add coconut oil. Once the oil is hot, add cumin seeds and almonds, fry well till almonds turn golden. Keep aside. Add onion and green chili and sauté well for 2-3 minutes. Add ginger-garlic paste and fry till the raw smell goes away. Now add eggplants, zucchinis pieces and fry for 3 minutes, then add tomatoes and fry till mushy. Add coriander powder, Garam masala, red chili powder, salt, and mix well. Fry for 2 minutes. Add rice and water, mix. Turn off Sauté mode, secure the lid and turn the vent to Sealing. Push the Rice button and natural pressure release. Garnish almonds and Cilantro if desired.

Nutrition Facts

Calories 537, Total Fat 18.4g, Saturated Fat 12.1g, Cholesterol 0mg, Sodium 103mg, Total Carbohydrate 84.2g, Dietary Fiber 4.2g, Total Sugars 4.8g, Protein 9.4g

Rosemary Rice with Cashews

Prep time: 10 min Cooking Time: 25 min serve: 2

Ingredients

1 bunches rosemary

1tablespoon coconut oil

½ teaspoon cumin seeds

½ teaspoon Garam masala

1 cup rice

2 cups water

¼ onion, sliced

1 tablespoon cashews

2 green chili, finely chopped

3 garlic pods, crushed

Salt to taste

Cilantro for garnishing

Instructions

Wash the rosemary bunch, make a fine paste of rosemary and green chili.

Press Sauté mode on High Pressure. Add coconut oil and let it get hot. Once hot, add cumin seeds and fry well. Add onions, garlic, and cashews, fry till golden. Add rosemary green chili paste and fry till raw smell goes away approximately 2-3 minutes. Add Garam masala, mix well. Add rice and water, add salt to taste. Mix gently. Turn off Sauté mode. Cover with the lid of Instant Pot and make sure the vent is set to Sealing. Push the Rice button. Quickly release once the Instant Pot goes to Warm mode or natural pressure release is also acceptable. 7. Fluff the rice and serve hot. Garnish with cilantro if desired.

Nutrition Facts

Calories 454, Total Fat 10.3g, Saturated Fat 4.7g, Cholesterol 16mg, Sodium 180mg, Total Carbohydrate 80.5g, Dietary Fiber 1.9g, Total Sugars 1.7g, Protein 8.3g

Cabbage Peas Rice

Prep time: 10 min Cooking Time: 20 min serve: 2

Ingredients

1 cup basmati rice

1 tablespoon coconut oil

1/8 teaspoon Asafoetida

¼ teaspoon mustard seeds

1/8 cup cashews

1/8 teaspoon turmeric

10 curry leaves

1 tablespoon ginger, grated

2 green chilies, minced

2 cups shredded cabbage

½ cup green peas

½ teaspoon salt

1 tablespoon orange juice

1/4 cup basil, chopped

1 1/2 tablespoon fresh coconut

Instructions

Rinse the rice 2-3 times, and then soak the rice in 2 cups of warm water for 2 hours. Drain the rice and keep it aside. Turn Instant Pot to Sauté mode. Once the —Hot‖ sign displays, add coconut oil and Asafoetida. Add mustard seeds and allow them to pop. Add cashews and sauté for a minute. Add turmeric, curry leaves, ginger, and green chili. Mix everything and cook until cashew is golden brown. Add grated cabbage, green peas, and salt. Mix again. Add drained rice and gently mix everything. Add 2 cups of water. Close Instant Pot lid with pressure valve to Sealing. Press the Rice button. Allow natural pressure release. Open Instant Pot and pour orange juice. Garnish with basil and coconut.

Enjoy hot!

Nutrition Facts

Calories 517, Total Fat 13.1g, Saturated Fat 7.7g, Cholesterol 0mg, Sodium 604mg, Total Carbohydrate

89g, Dietary Fiber 6.5g, Total Sugars 5.2g, Protein 11.5g

Vegetable Buckwheat

Prep time: 10 min Cooking Time: 20 min serve: 2

Ingredients

1 1/2 cups water

½ cup buckwheat

1 tablespoon avocado oil

1 small red onion, chopped

½ small green bell pepper, chopped

½ teaspoon garlic powder

1/8 teaspoon red pepper flakes

3 leeks, thinly sliced

1 1/2 tablespoons soy sauce

½ cup green peas

½ teaspoon soy sauce

1 carrot

1/4 cup roasted peanuts

Instructions

Turn Instant Pot to Sauté mode. Once the —Hot‖ sign displays, add avocado oil.

Add red onions, green bell pepper, garlic powder, and pepper flakes to taste. Cook 3 minutes.

Add buckwheat, leeks, green peas, carrot, and soy sauce. Add 1 1/2 cups of water.

Close Instant Pot lid with pressure valve to Sealing. Press the Rice button. Allow natural pressure release. Open Instant Pot. Garnish with roasted peanuts.

Enjoy hot!

Nutrition Facts

Calories 455, Total Fat 11.9g, Saturated Fat 1.8g, Cholesterol 0mg, Sodium 512mg, Total Carbohydrate

73.3g, Dietary Fiber 9.8g, Total Sugars 12.8g, Protein 13.9g

Asparagus and Kale Risotto

Prep time: 10 min Cooking Time: 25 min serve: 2

Ingredients

2 tablespoon coconut oil, divided

1 small onion, chopped

1/2 cup Arborio rice

1/2 cup asparagus

¼ cup green peas

2 cups vegetable broth

1/4 teaspoon salt

2 cups kale

1/4 cup grated goat cheese

Instructions

Select Sauté, add 1 tablespoon of coconut oil to the inner pot. When it has stopped foaming, add the onion and cook, stirring, until the onion pieces separate and soften about 3 minutes. Add the rice and stir to coat in the coconut oil, cooking for about 1 minute. Stir in the asparagus, green peas. Stirring for 2-3 minutes.

Add stock and the salt, and stir to combine. Lock the lid into place. Select Pressure Cook or Manual, and adjust the pressure to High and the time to 8 minutes. After cooking, quickly release the pressure.

Unlock the lid. Test the onion; the rice should be soft with a slightly athletic center, and the sauce should be creamy, but it will probably not be entirely done. Add kale. Select Sauté and adjust to Medium heat. Simmer for 2-3 minutes until the kale is wilted and the sauce is creamy. Stir in the cheese. Taste and adjust the seasoning. Serve.

Nutrition Facts

Calories 411, Total Fat 16.6g, Saturated Fat 13.1g, Cholesterol 4mg, Sodium 1101mg, Total

Carbohydrate 53g, Dietary Fiber 4.7g, Total Sugars 3.9g, Protein 13.2g

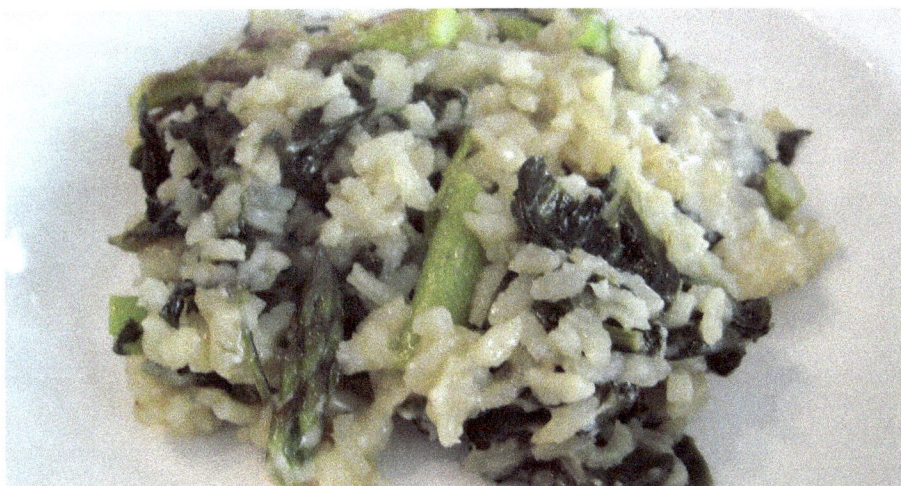

Soups and Salads

Borlotti Bean Soup

Ingredients

1 pound borlotti beans, sorted and rinsed

2 quarts veggie stock

1 medium red onion, diced

5 cloves of garlic, peeled and smashed

2 tsp. sea salt

1/4 tsp white pepper

2 medium sweet potatoes, diced

1 pound frozen, sliced parsnips

3/4 cup chopped sun-dried tomatoes*

1-2 tsp dried dill

3-4 tbsp fresh, minced parsley

Directions:

Place the beans, stock, onion, garlic, sea salt, and pepper in a pot. Cook them over low-medium heat. Simmer for 3-4 hours, or longer, add water as needed. As the beans become soft, add the sweet potato and simmer until the potatoes become tender. Add the carrots, tomatoes, and dill. Cook the parsnips until heated thoroughly. Add the parsley, season with additional salt and white pepper.

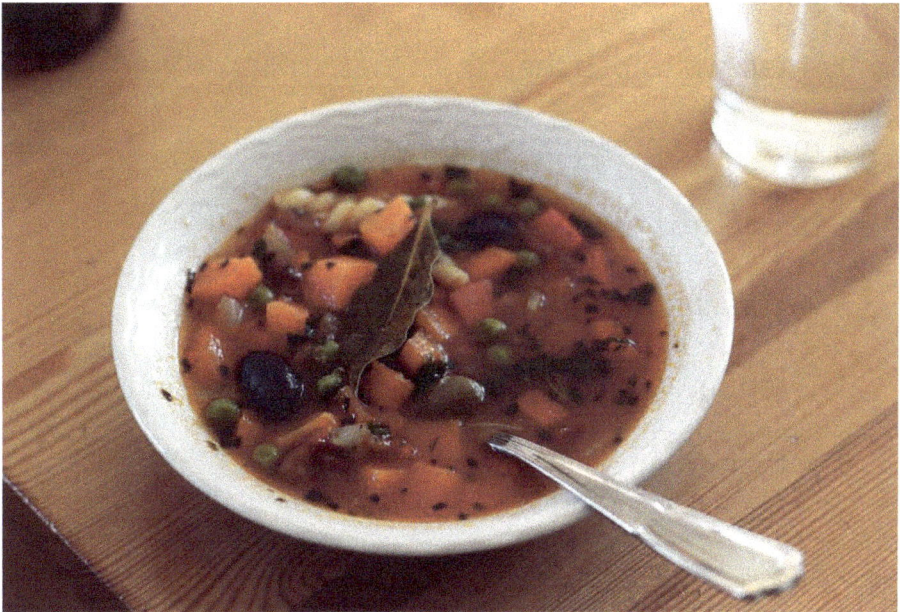

Lentil Soup

Ingredients

1/2 pound lentils, sorted and rinsed

½ pound fava beans sorted and rinsed

2 quarts veggie broth

1 medium red onion, diced

6 cloves of garlic, peeled and smashed

2 tsp. sea salt

1/4 tsp white pepper

2 medium potatoes, diced

1 pound frozen, sliced carrots

3/4 cup chopped sun-dried tomatoes*

1-2 tsp dried dill

3-4 tbsp fresh, minced parsley

Directions:

Place the beans, broth, red onion, garlic, sea salt, and pepper in a pot. Cook them over low-medium heat.

Simmer for 3-4 hours, or longer, add water as needed. As the beans become soft, add the potato and simmer until the potatoes become tender. Add the carrots, tomatoes, and dill. Cook the carrots until heated thoroughly. Add the parsley, season with additional salt and white pepper.

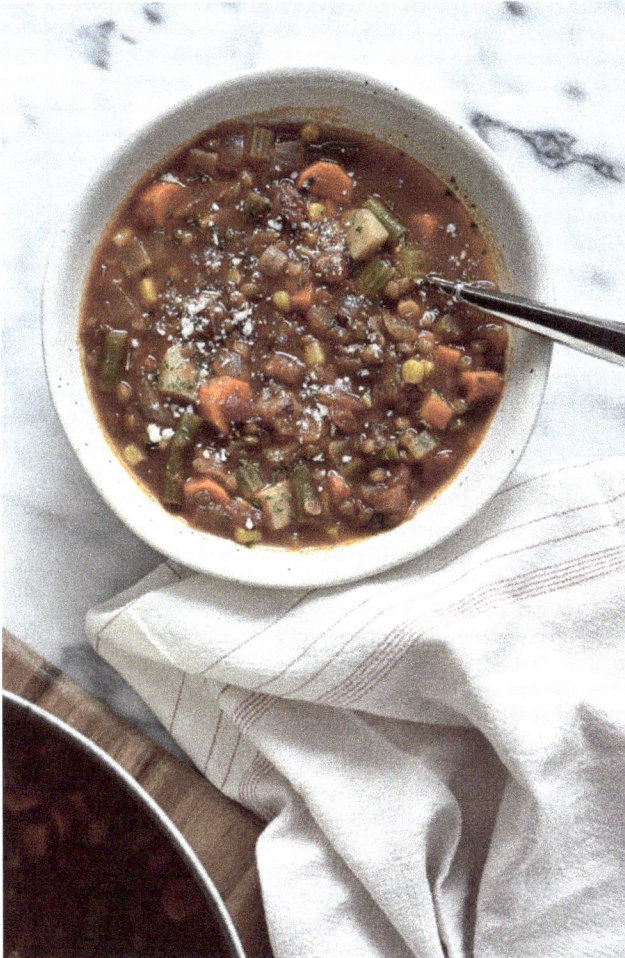

Triple Bean Soup

Ingredients

1/2 pound borlotti beans, sorted and rinsed

¼ pound great northern beans, sorted and rinsed

¼ pound kidney beans sorted and rinsed

2 quarts veggie broth

1 medium onion, diced

5 cloves of garlic, peeled and smashed

2 tsp. sea salt

1/4 tsp rainbow peppercorns

2 medium potatoes, diced

1 pound frozen, sliced carrots

3/4 cup chopped sun-dried tomatoes*

1-2 tsp dried dill

3-4 tbsp fresh, minced parsley

Directions:

Place the beans, stock, onion, garlic, sea salt, and pepper in a pot. Cook them over low-medium heat. Simmer for 3-4 hours, or longer, add water as needed. As the beans become soft, add the potato and simmer until the potatoes become tender. Add the carrots, tomatoes, and dill. Cook the carrots until heated thoroughly. Add the parsley, season with additional salt and peppercorns.

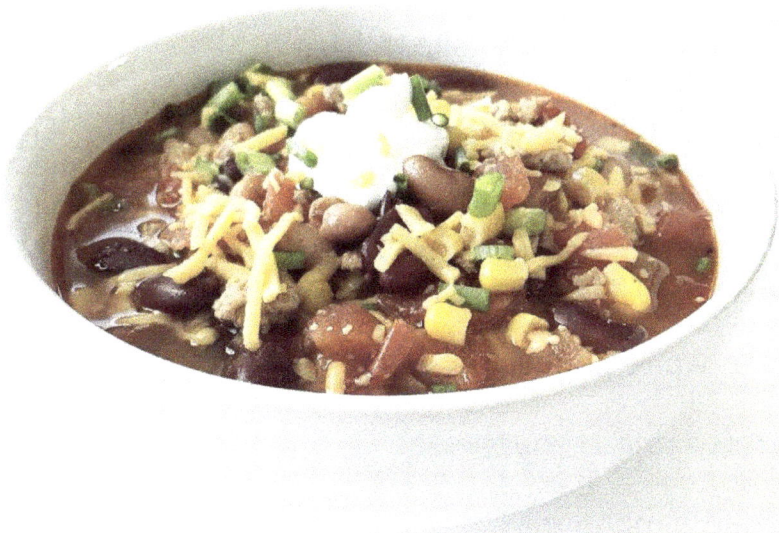

Parsnips and Summer Squash Soup

Ingredients

1 medium summer squash (1 lb of peeled and cubed butternut squash)

1/2 medium red onion, diced

½ medium yellow onion, diced

2/3 lb parsnips, peeled and cut into chunks

1 carrot, peeled and sliced

3 cups vegetable broth

1 bay leaf

1 tsp sea salt

1 tsp white pepper

1/4 tsp dried ground sage

½ can almond milk

Directions:

Combine the squash, red and yellow onion, parsnips, apple, broth, and bay leaf in a slow cooker. Cover and cook on low for about 6 hours or until veggies are soft. Take out the bay leaf and discard. Transfer these ingredients to a blender and blend until smooth Pour it back to the slow cooker, season with salt, pepper & sage. Pour the almond milk. Add more salt and pepper to taste.

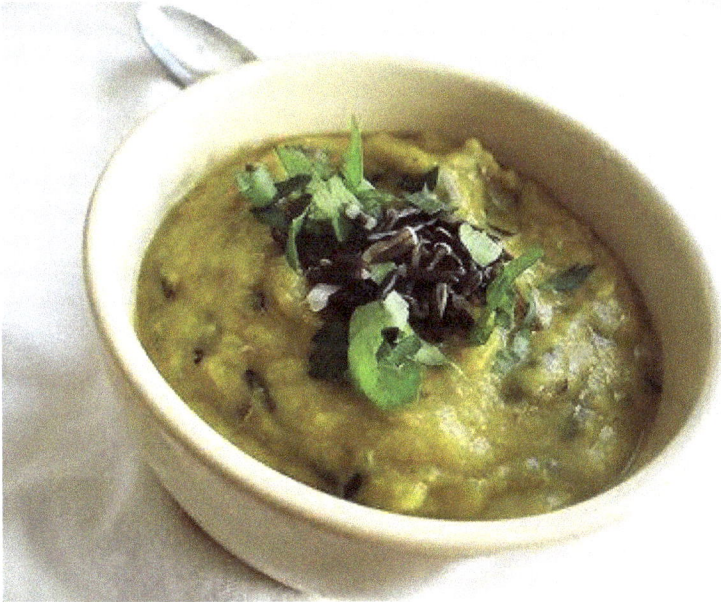

Butternut Squash and Apple Soup

Ingredients

1 medium butternut squash (1 lb of peeled and cubed butternut squash)

1 medium red onion, diced

2/3 lb parsnips, peeled and cut into chunks

1 Washington apple, peeled and sliced

3 cups vegetable stock

1 bay leaf

1 tsp sea salt

1 tsp white pepper

1/4 tsp dried ground sage

½ can use coconut milk

Directions:

Combine the squash, red onion, carrots, apple, stock, and bay leaf in a slow cooker. Cover and cook on low for about 6 hours or until veggies are soft. Take out the bay leaf and discard. Transfer these ingredients to a blender and blend until smooth Pour it back to the slow cooker, season with sea salt, pepper & sage. Pour the coconut milk.

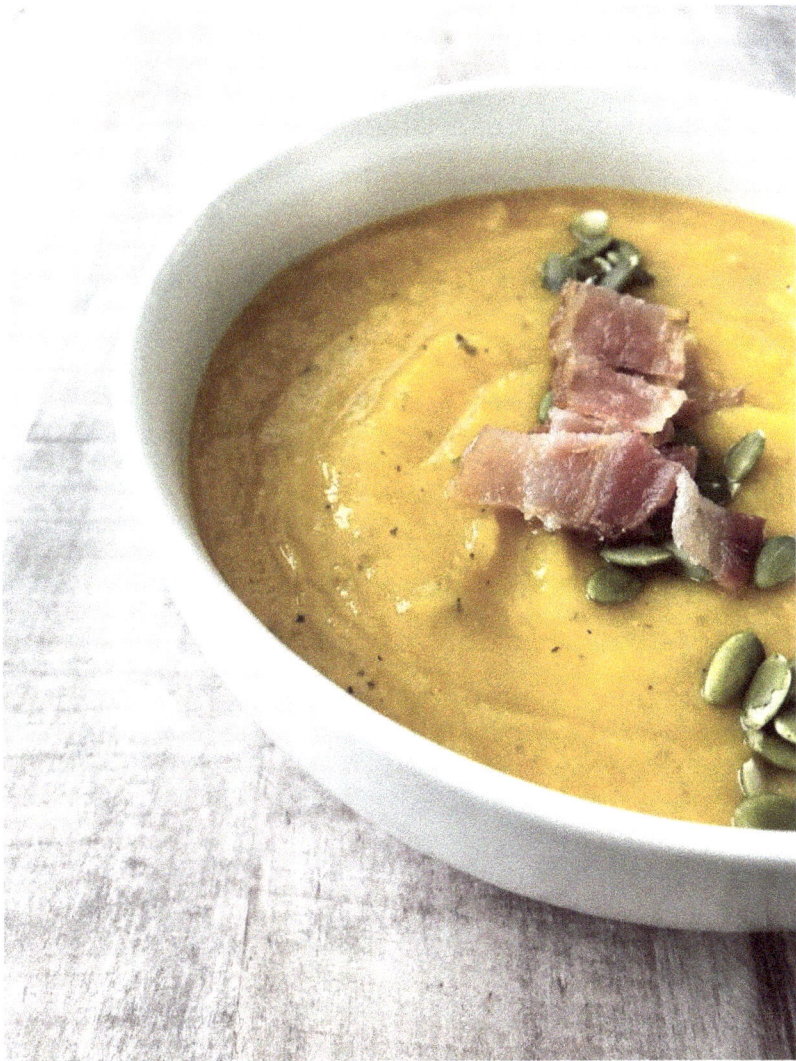

Avocado and Lima Bean Salad Sandwich

Ingredients

1 15-oz. can lima beans, rinsed, drained, and skinned

1 large, ripe avocado

1/4 cup chopped fresh cilantro

2 Tbsp. chopped green onions Juice of

1 lime Sea salt and pepper, to taste Bread of your
choice

Directions:

Lettuce Tomato Mash the lima beans and avocado with
a fork. Add cilantro, green onions, and lime juice and
stir. Season with salt and pepper. Spread on your
favorite bread and garnish with lettuce and tomato

Rice Noodle Salad with Chili Garlic Sauce

Ingredients

Sauce:

3 tbsp Soy Sauce

1 tbsp Rice Wine Vinegar

1 tbsp Honey 1 tsp. chili garlic sauce

6 tbsp. canola oil

Salad:

100 g Rice Noodles

1 Carrot

1 Zucchini

1/4 Purple Cabbage finely sliced

1 Green Bell Pepper finely sliced

1 Yellow Pepper finely sliced

1 bunch Fresh Coriander roughly chopped

1 small handful Cashew Nuts roughly chopped

1 tsp Sesame Seeds

1/2 Red Chili Combine all of the sauce ingredients.

Soak the noodles according to the instructions in the packaging.

Directions:

 Combine with carrots and zucchini. Add all of the remaining finely chopped veggies in. Combine with the sauce, and garnish with the coriander, cashews, sesame seeds, and chili.

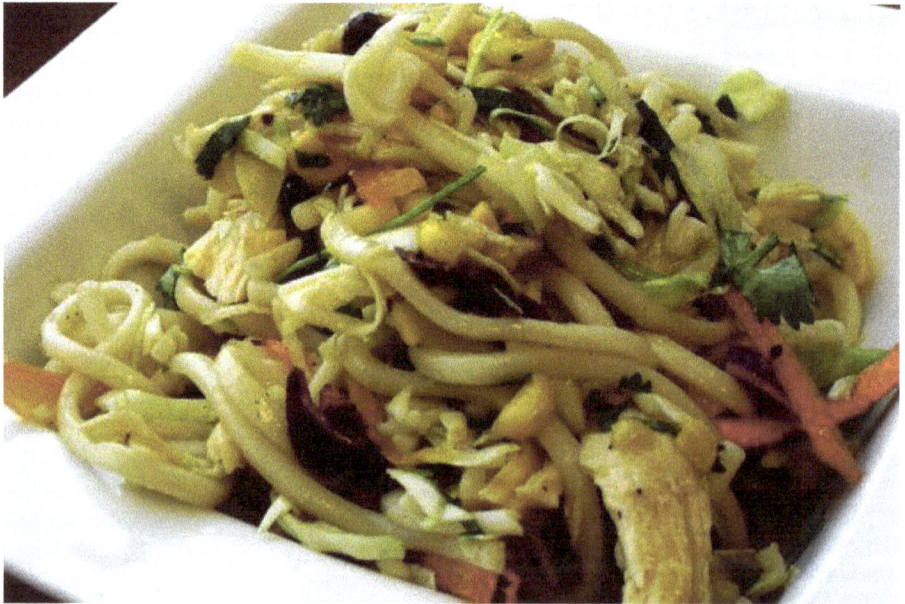

Bib Lettuce and Vegan Ricotta Salad

Ingredients:

6 to 7 cups bib lettuce,

3 bundles, trimmed

1/4 cucumber, halved lengthwise, then thinly sliced

16 grapes

1/2 cup sliced almonds

1/4 white onion, sliced

Salt and pepper, to taste

3 ounces mozzarella cheese, shredded

3 ounces parmesan cheese, shredded

1 ounce blue cheese, crumbled

Dressing:

1 tablespoon distilled white vinegar

1/4 lemon, juiced, about

Two teaspoons

1/4 cup extra-virgin olive oil

1 tbsp. Chimichurri sauce Prep Combine all of the dressing ingredients in a food processor.

Directions:

Toss with the rest of the ingredients and combine well.

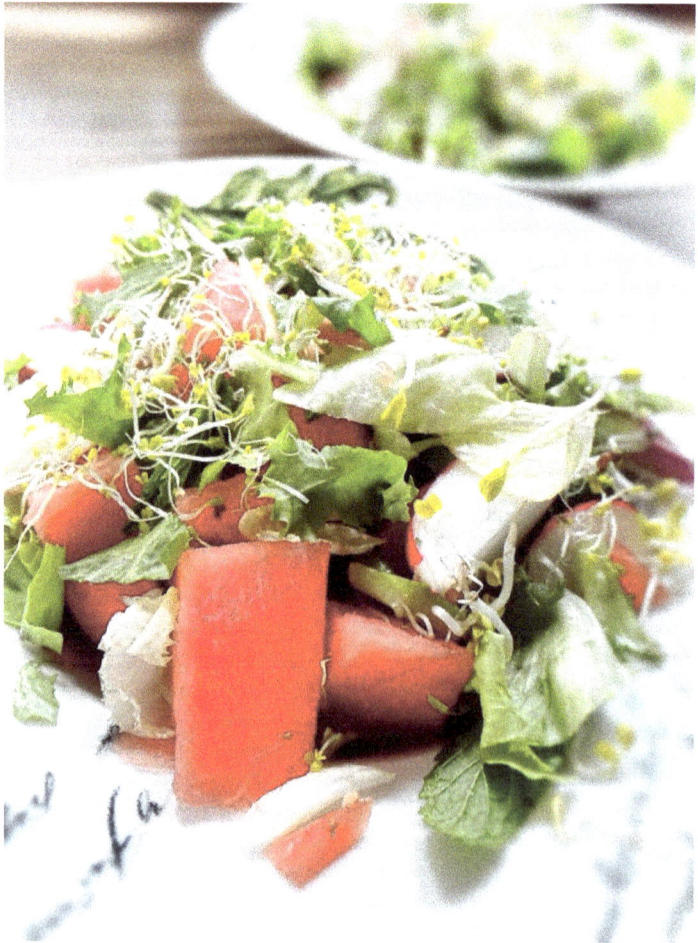

Endive Lettuce Tomatillo and Vegan Ricotta Salad

Ingredients:

6 to 7 cups endive,

3 bundles, trimmed

1/4 cucumber, halved lengthwise, then thinly sliced

3 tablespoons chopped or snipped chives

16 green tomatillos, sliced in half

1/2 cup sliced almonds

1/4 white onion, sliced Salt, and pepper, to taste

3 ounces pecorino romano cheese, shredded

3 ounces cream cheese, crumbled

3 ounces Camembert cheese, crumbled Dressing

1 tablespoon distilled white vinegar

1/4 lemon, juiced, about 2 teaspoons

1/4 cup extra-virgin olive oil

1 tsp. Dijon mustard

Directions:

Combine all of the dressing ingredients in a food processor. Toss with the rest of the ingredients and combine well.

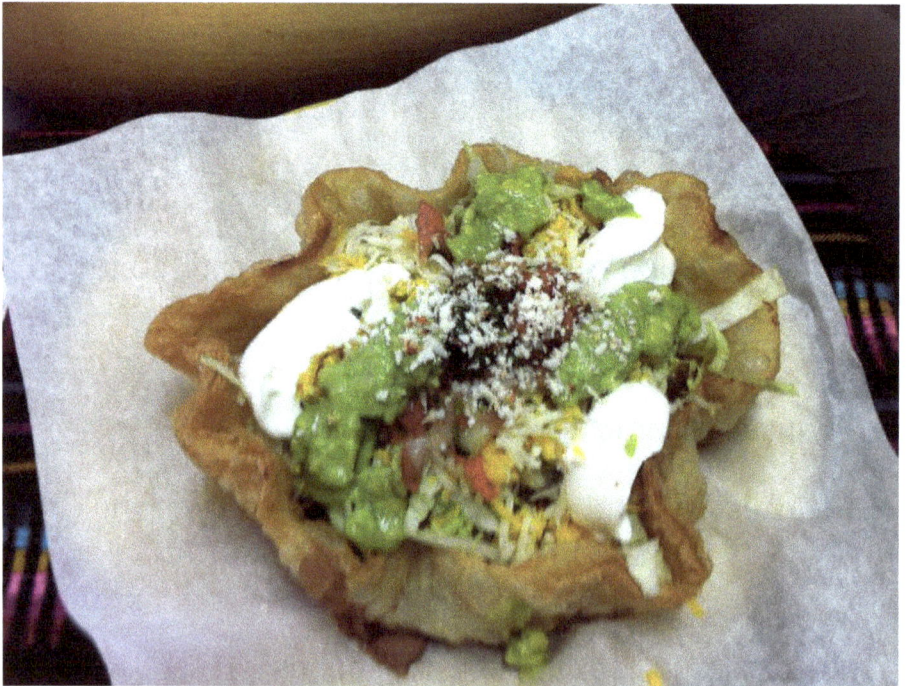

Dinner

Creamy Cilantro Lime Coleslaw

This creamy cilantro lime coleslaw is a delicious low carb side dish that is perfect for summer picnics or to serve alongside tacos or anything on the grill. This slaw is not only crunchy and cream, but th lime and cilantro add so much flavor! Each serving is only 3.2g net carbs

Prep Time 10 minutes Total Time 10 minutes Servings 5

Ingredients

14 oz coleslaw, bagged 1 1/2 avocados

1/4 cup cilantro leaves 2 limes, juiced

1 garlic clove 1/4 cup water

1/2 teaspoon salt cilantro to garnish

Instructions

In a food processor add the garlic and cilantro and process until chopped. Add the lime juice, avocados and water. Pulse until nice and creamy. Take out the avocado mixture and in a large bowl mix it with the coleslaw. It will be a bit thick but it will cover the slaw nicely. For best results, refrigerate for a few hours before eating to soften the cabbage.

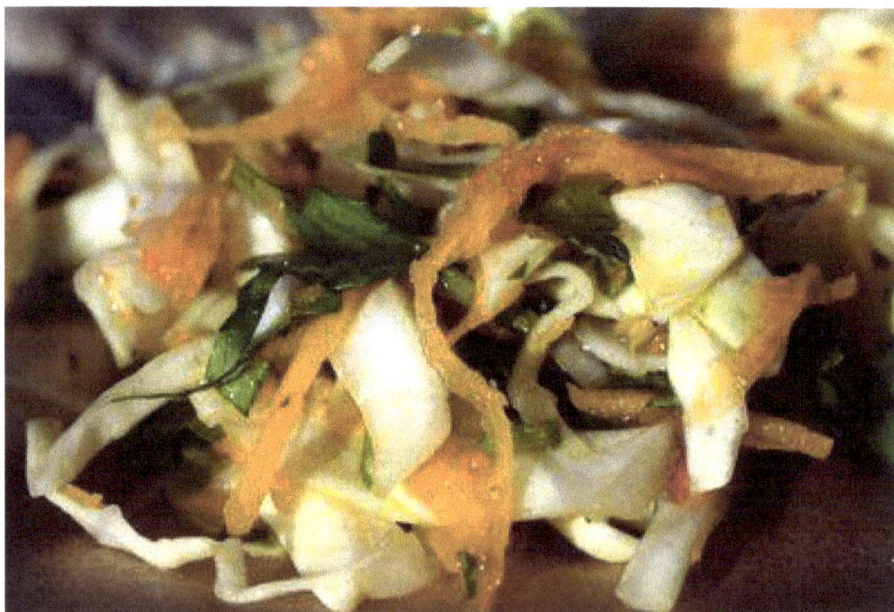

Fried Goat Cheese

Total Time 13 minutes Servings 8 servings Prep Time: 10 minutes Cook Time: 3 minutes

Ingredients:

1 oz pork rinds, finely ground

8 ounce (package) goat cheese log, cold

2 large eggs

1/2 tsp Dried Parsley

1/4 tsp Pink Himalayan Salt 1/2 cup Coconut flour

1 1/2 cup Coconut Oil (For Cooking)

Instructions:

Add coconut oil to a small saucepan and heat on medium-high heat. Place a thermometer in the oil to keep track of temp.

Place coconut flour in a small bowl, whisk two eggs into a second bowl and add the ground pork finely to a third bowl. You can easily grind the pork rinds by adding to a zip top bag and crush them.

Cut the 8 ounce log into 8 even pieces and place on a plate. One at a time coat the goat cheese in coconut flour, egg wash and then pork rinds and place back onto the plate.

When the coconut oil has reached 345 degrees add two goat cheese to the oil and cook for 30 seconds. Gently flip and cook for an additional 30 seconds. Remove and set on a plate with a paper towel.

Repeat until all goat cheese has been fried. Serve with favorite dipping sauce and enjoy!

NOTE: we find keeping the oil between 330 and 350 degrees is the best for frying. You can do this by turning the heat up and down as you see fit.

Nutrition Info

Calories 114 Calories from Fat 67 Fat 7.4g
Carbohydrates 3g Fiber 1.25g

Protein 8.25g

Easy Cheesy Zucchini Gratin

This Easy Cheesy Zucchini Gratin has become a staple in our house! It's cheesy and creamy, super easy to throw together, and the perfect low carb side dish for your keto diet!

Prep Time: 10 minutes Cook Time: 46 minutes Total Time: 56 minutes Servings: 9 servings

Ingredients

4 cups sliced raw zucchini

1 small onion, peeled and sliced thin salt and pepper to taste

1 1/2 cups shredded pepper jack cheese 2 Tbsp butter

1/2 tsp garlic powder

1/2 cup heavy whipping cream 1/4 teaspoon xanthan gum

Instructions

Preheat oven to 375 degrees (F).

Grease a 9×9 or equivalent oven proof pan.

Overlap 1/3 of the zucchini and onion slices in the pan, then season with salt and pepper and sprinkle with 1/2 cup of shredded cheese.

Repeat two more times until you have three layers and have used up all of the zucchini, onions, and shredded cheese.

Combine the garlic powder, butter, heavy cream, and xanthan gum in a microwave safe dish.

Heat for one minute or until the butter has melted. Whisk until smooth.

Gently pour the butter and cream mixture over the zucchini layers.

Bake at 375 degrees (F) for about 45 minutes, or until the liquid has thickened and the top is golden brown.

Serve warm.

Nutrition Info

Serving Size: 3 x 3 square Calories: 230 Fat: 20g

Carbohydrates: 3g net Protein: 8g

Low Carb Cauliflower Rice Mushroom Risotto

Prep Time: 20 minutes Cook Time: 30 minutes Total Time: 50 minutes Servings: 6

Ingredients

1   tablespoons butter

2 tablespoons olive oil 6 cloves garlic, minced 1 small onion, diced

1 large shallot, minced

8 ounces cremini mushrooms, thinly sliced 2 cup chicken stock, divided

4 cups riced cauliflower 1 cup heavy cream

½ cup grated Parmesan cheese

2 tablespoons chopped fresh flat-leaf parsley Sea salt and black pepper, to taste

Instructions

In a large sauté pan, heat the butter and olive oil over medium heat. To the pan, add the garlic, onion, and shallot. Sauté until the onions are soft and translucent and the garlic is fragrant. About 5 minutes.

To the pan, add the mushrooms and 1 cup chicken stock. Sauté until mushrooms are soft and have released their liquid. About 5 minutes.

Add the cauliflower and remaining 1 cup of chicken stock and stirring frequently, sauté for 10 minutes.

Reduce the heat to low, stir in the heavy cream, Parmesan cheese, parsley, salt and pepper. Let simmer for 10 to 15 minutes to thicken.

Nutrition Info

Calories: 297 Fat: 26g

Carbohydrates: Net 7.5g Protein: 7g

Spinach and Mushroom Breakfast Casserole

Prep Time 15 mins Cook Time 45 mins Total Time 1 hr
Servings 12

Ingredients

5 Tablespoons unsalted butter divided

1 medium onion chopped (about 7 ounces) 8 ounces mushrooms sliced

12 ounce baby spinach 2 cloves garlic minced 6 eggs beaten

16 oz. cottage cheese

12 ounces sharp cheddar cheese grated 3 green onions sliced

1 teaspoon kosher salt

1/2 teaspoon black pepper

Instructions

Pre-heat oven to 350* F. Use 1 Tablespoon butter to grease 13" X 9" baking dish.

Heat 4 Tablespoons butter in a large skillet or sauté pan, and sauté yellow onions and mushrooms, about 3-4 of minutes until onions are translucent and mushrooms are soft. Add garlic and sauté another minute.

Add spinach, a handful at a time, and sauté. Cover skillet and let spinach wilt, about 5 minutes.

Let cool, drain excess liquid, and chop more finely.

In a separate bowl, whisk eggs, cottage cheese, cheddar cheese, green onions, and salt and pepper. Add cooked spinach and mushroom mixture.

Mix well and pour into baking dish.

Bake for 45-50 minutes or until top is golden brown and center is done.

Nutrition Info

Calories: 241kcal Carbohydrates: 5g Protein: 16g

Fat: 18g

Saturated Fat: 10g Cholesterol: 131mg Sodium: 564mg Potassium: 337mg Fiber: 1g Sugar: 2g

Grilled Kale and Romaine Lettuce

Ingredients

1 bunch of Kale

1 bunch of Romaine Lettuce leaves

1 winter squash, peeled and sliced lengthwise

1/3 cup Italian parsley or basil, finely chopped

Dressing:

6 tbsp. extra virgin olive oil

Sea salt, to taste

3 tbsp. Balsamic vinegar

Directions:

Dijon mustard Combine all of the dressing ingredients thoroughly. Preheat your grill to low heat and grease the grates. Layer the vegetable grill for 12 minutes per side until tender, flipping once. Brush with the marinade/ dressing ingredients

Grilled Okra and Endives

Ingredients

10 pcs. Okra

1 bunch of endives

1/3 cup Italian parsley or basil, finely chopped

Dressing:

6 tbsp. olive oil

3 dashes of Tabasco hot sauce

Sea salt, to taste

3 tbsp. white wine vinegar

Directions:

Egg-free mayonnaise Combine all of the dressing ingredients thoroughly. Preheat your grill to low heat and grease the grates. Layer the vegetable grill for 12 minutes per side until tender, flipping once. Brush with the marinade/ dressing ingredients

Grilled Rutabaga Edamame Beans and Cabbage

Ingredients

20 pcs. Edamame Beans

1 medium Cabbage sliced

1 medium Rutabaga, peeled and cut in half lengthwise

2 medium carrots, cut lengthwise and cut in half

4 large Tomatoes, sliced thick

1/3 cup Italian parsley or basil, finely chopped

Dressing:

6 tbsp. olive oil

3 dashes of Tabasco hot sauce

Sea salt, to taste

3 tbsp. white wine vinegar

Directions:

Egg-free mayonnaise Combine all of the dressing ingredients thoroughly. Preheat your grill to low heat and grease the grates. Layer the vegetable grill for 12 minutes per side until tender, flipping once. Brush with the marinade/ dressing ingredients

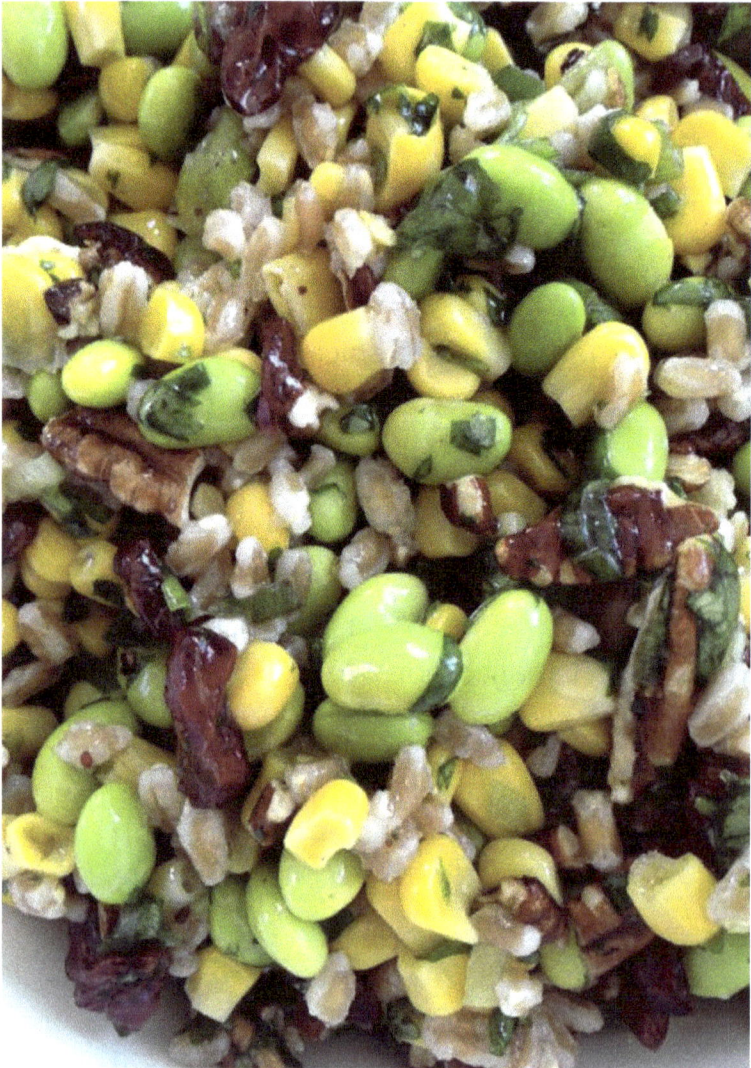

Grilled Summer Squash Beets and Artichoke Hearts

Ingredients

5 pcs. Beets 1 cup artichoke hearts

1 bunch of Romaine Lettuce leaves

1 butternut squash, peeled and sliced lengthwise

4 large Tomatoes, sliced thick

Dressing:

6 tbsp. olive oil

3 dashes of Tabasco hot sauce

Sea salt, to taste

3 tbsp. white wine vinegar

Directions:

Egg-free mayonnaise Combine all of the dressing ingredients thoroughly. Preheat your grill to low heat and grease the grates. Layer the vegetable grill for 12 minutes per side until tender, flipping once. Brush with the marinade/ dressing ingredients

Grilled Button and Shitake Mushroom

Ingredients

12 oz. fresh button mushrooms

4 oz. shiitake mushrooms

1 bunch of collard greens

4 tablespoons canola oil, divided

Sea salt and freshly ground black pepper

2 tablespoons reduced-sodium soy sauce

2 tablespoons unseasoned rice vinegar

1 tablespoon toasted sesame oil

1 teaspoon finely grated peeled ginger

6 scallions, thinly sliced on a diagonal

2 teaspoons toasted sesame seeds

Directions:

Combine the mushrooms and carrots with 3 Tbsp. Canola oil in a bowl. Season with salt and pepper. Grill while turning the mushrooms and carrots frequently until tender. Combine the soy sauce, vinegar, sesame oil, ginger, and remaining 1 Tbsp. Canola oil in a bowl. Cut the carrots into 2 inch long pieces. Cut the mushrooms into bite-size pieces. Combine them with the vinaigrette, scallions, and sesame seeds. Season with salt and pepper.

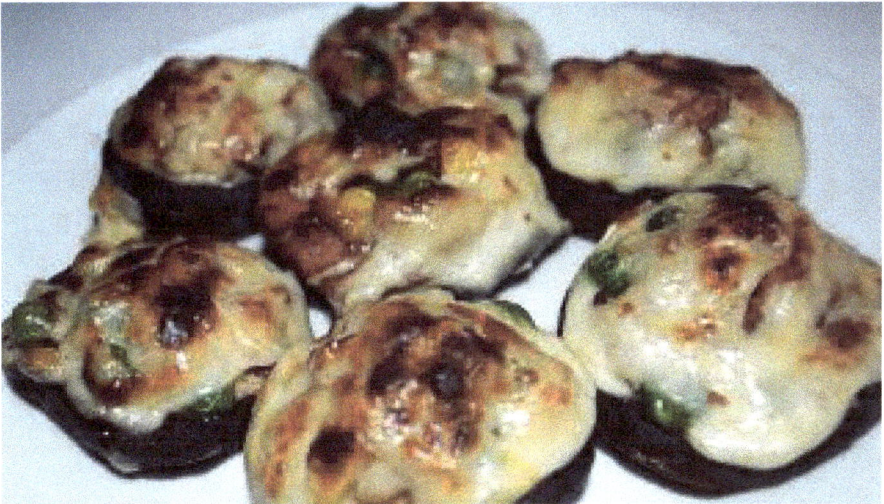

Sweets

Almond Banana Chocolate Muffins
Prep time: 15 min Cooking Time: 30 min serve: 2

Ingredients

1 banana

1 cup water

1 egg

¼ tablespoon coconut oil

¼ teaspoon applesauce

½ cup almond flour

1 tablespoon honey

¼ teaspoon baking powder

¼ teaspoon baking soda

½ cup sliced California almonds, divided

½ cup semi-sweet chocolate chips

Instructions

In a large bowl, stir together banana, almond flour, baking powder, baking soda and honey. Stir in coconut oil, applesauce and egg; chocolate chips and almond mix well. Pour batter into prepared muffin cups.

Pour 1 cup water into the Instant Pot. Place the trivet inside. Place the muffin cups on the rack or pan.

Press the Pressure Cook or Manual button and set the cook time to 20 minutes.

When the Instant Pot beeps, allow the pressure to release naturally for 10 minutes, then carefully switch the Pressure Release valve to Venting. When fully released, open the lid. Carefully remove the muffins.

Nutrition Facts

Calories 165, Total Fat 10.6g, Saturated Fat 2g Cholesterol 41mg , Sodium 29mg, Total Carbohydrate

12.3g, Dietary Fiber 2.8g , Total Sugars 5.7g, Protein 5.1g

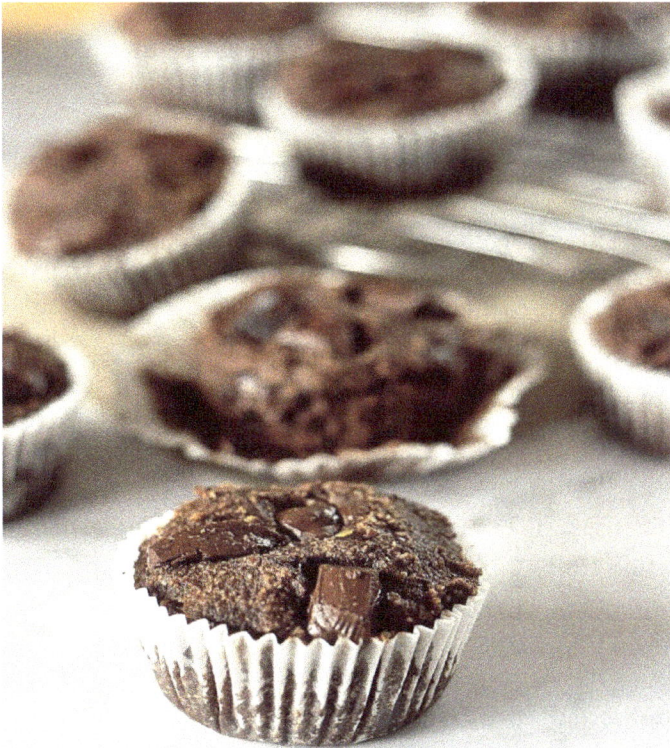

Cinnamon Bran Muffins

Prep time: 15 min Cooking Time: 30 min serve: 2

Ingredients

1/2 cup bran flakes cereal

1 cup coconut flour

½ tablespoon honey

½ teaspoon baking powder

½ teaspoon ground cinnamon

½ cup buttermilk

1/2 tablespoon butter, melted

½ teaspoon vanilla extract

1 cup water

Instructions

In a large bowl, combine bran flakes, coconut flour, honey, baking powder and cinnamon. Stir in buttermilk, butter, and vanilla. Spoon mixture into prepared muffin cups.

Pour 1 cup water into the Instant Pot. Place the trivet inside. Place the muffin cups on the rack or pan.

Secure the lid and set the Pressure Release valve to Sealing. Press the Pressure Cook or Manual button and set the cook time to 20 minutes.

When the Instant Pot beeps, allow the pressure to release naturally for 10 minutes, then carefully switch the

Pressure Release valve to Venting. When fully released, open the lid. Carefully remove the muffins.

Nutrition Facts

Calories 65, Total Fat 2.3g, Saturated Fat 1.6g, Cholesterol 5mg, Sodium 61mg, Total Carbohydrate 9g, Dietary Fiber 2.1g, Total Sugars 4.3g, Protein 2.1g

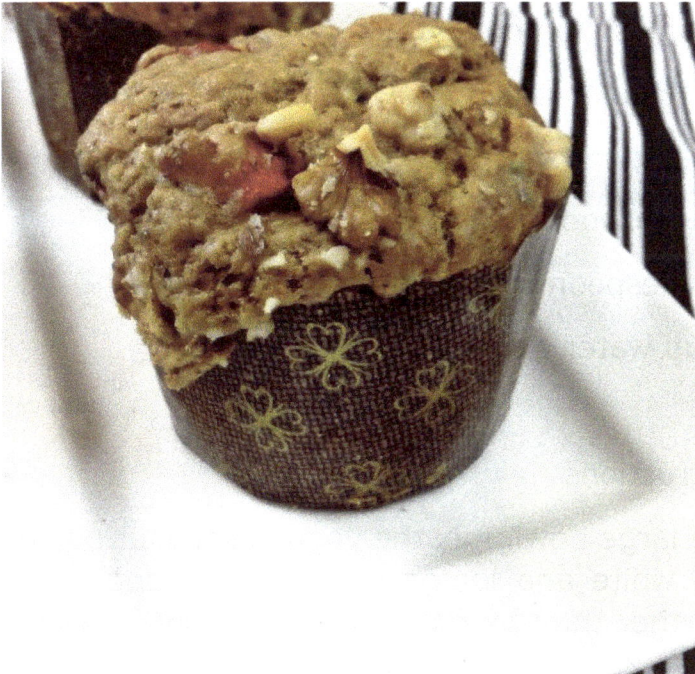

Raspberry Lemon Muffins

Prep time: 15 min Cooking Time: 15 min serve: 2

Ingredients

½ tablespoon plain yogurt

1 tablespoon coconut oil

½ tablespoon lemon juice

1 egg white

½ teaspoon lemon extract

½ cup flax meal

½ tablespoon honey

¼ teaspoon baking powder

¼ teaspoon salt

1/8 teaspoon grated lemon zest

1 tablespoon frozen raspberries

1 cup water

Instructions

In a large bowl, mix the yogurt, coconut oil, lemon juice, egg white and lemon extract. In a separate bowl, stir together the flax meal, honey, baking powder, salt, and lemon zest. Add the wet ingredients to the dry, and mix until just blended. Gently stir in the frozen raspberries. Spoon batter evenly into the prepared muffin cups.

Pour 1 cup water into the Instant Pot. Place the trivet inside. Place the muffin cups on the rack or pan.

Secure the lid and set the Pressure Release valve to Sealing. Press the Pressure Cook or Manual button and set the cook time to 20 minutes.

When the Instant Pot beeps, allow the pressure to release naturally for 10 minutes, then carefully switch the Pressure Release valve to Venting. When fully released, open the lid. Carefully remove the muffins.

Nutrition Facts

Calories 123, Total Fat 8.5g, Saturated Fat 3g, Cholesterol 0mg , Sodium 158mg, Total Carbohydrate

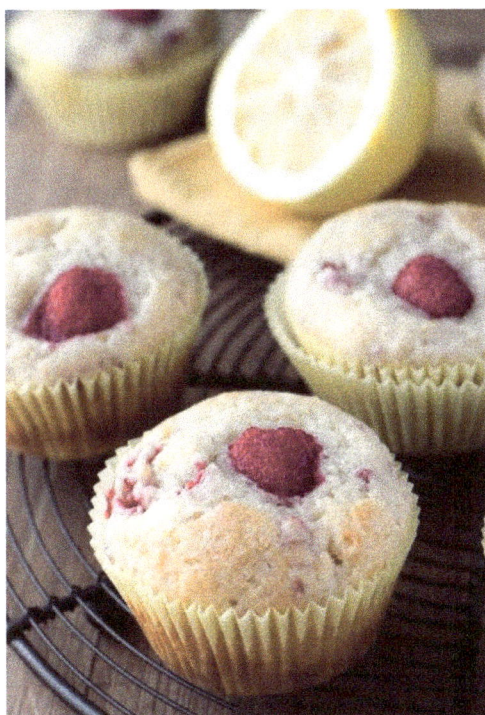

Blackberry Peach Muffins

Prep time: 15 min Cooking Time: 20 min serve: 2

Ingredients

½ cup coconut flour

1 tablespoon honey

½ teaspoon baking powder

1 pinch salt

1 egg

¼ cup coconut milk

½ tablespoon melted butter

¼ cup blackberries

1/8 cup peeled and diced fresh peaches

¼ teaspoon ground cinnamon

1/8 teaspoon ground nutmeg

1 cup water

Instructions

In a large bowl, stir together the coconut flour, honey, baking powder and salt. In a separate bowl, mix the egg, coconut milk, cinnamon, nutmeg and ½ cup of melted butter until well blended. Pour the wet ingredients into the dry, and mix until just blended. Fold in the blackberries and peaches. Fill muffin cups with batter.

Pour 1 cup water into the Instant Pot. Place the trivet inside. Place the muffin cups on the rack or pan.

Secure the lid and set the Pressure Release valve to Sealing. Press the Pressure Cook or Manual button and set the cook time to 20 minutes.

When the Instant Pot beeps, allow the pressure to release naturally for 10 minutes, then carefully switch the Pressure Release valve to Venting. When fully released, open the lid. Carefully remove the muffins.

Nutrition Facts

Calories 145, Total Fat 7.7g, Saturated Fat 5.4g, Cholesterol 45mg, Sodium 68mg, Total Carbohydrate 16.9g, Dietary Fiber 7g, Total Sugars 5.6g, Protein 3.9g

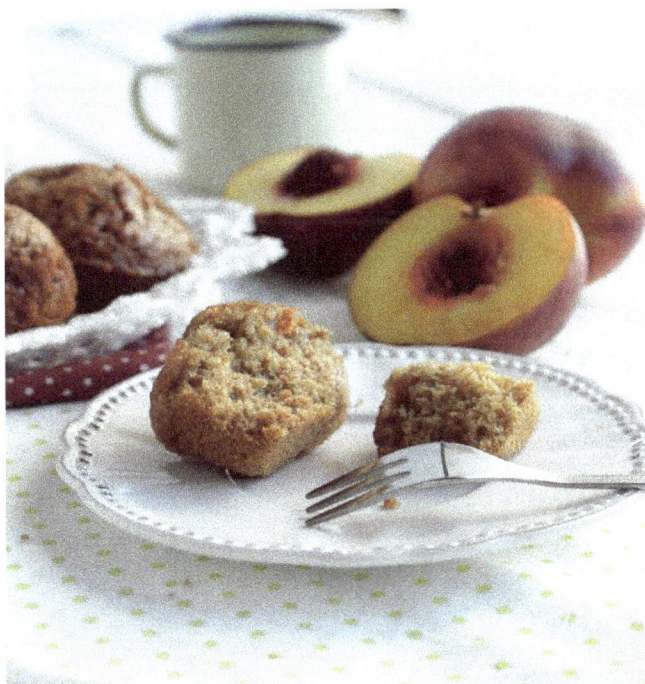

No-bake keto granola bars with peanut butter

No-bake keto granola bars peanut butter, easy healthy granola bars. Creamy peanut butter, flaxseed meal, chia seeds, almonds, coconut and more! 100% Sugar free, gluten free paleo breakfast or snacks.

Prep Time: 10 mins Total Time: 30 mins

Servings: 8 breakfast bars

Ingredients

Wet ingredients

1/2 cup Natural Peanut butter or almond butter if paleo 1/4 cup Coconut oil

2 teaspoons Vanilla extract Dry ingredients

1/3 cup Erythritol - like erythritol

1/2 cup Sliced almonds + extra 1 tablespoon to decorate on top 1/3 cup Flaxseed meal

1 tablespoon Chia seeds 1/3 cup Pumpkin seeds

1/4 cup Unsweetened desiccated Coconut 1/2 teaspoon Cinnamon

Chocolate drizzle

3 tablespoons Sugar-free Chocolate Chips 1 teaspoon Coconut oil

Instructions

Line a loaf pan, size 9 inches x 5 inches, with parchment paper. Set aside.

In a medium mixing bowl or a saucepan, place all the wet ingredients: peanut butter, coconut oil, and vanilla.

Microwave by 30 seconds burst, stir and repeat until the coconut oil is fully melted and combines with the nut butter. It should not take more than 1 minute 30 seconds. Otherwise, melt the ingredients in a saucepan under medium heat, stirring often to prevent the mixture from sticking to the pan.

Stir in the sugar-free crystal sweetener, stir and microwave an extra 30 seconds to incorporate well. Erythritol doesn't dissolve very well but it will give some delicious sweet crunch into your bars or see paleo note.

In a large mixing bowl, add the rest of the dry ingredients: sliced almonds, flaxseed meal, chia seeds, pumpkin seeds, shredded coconut, and cinnamon. Stir to combine.

Pour the nut butter mixture onto the dry ingredients. Stir with a spatula to combine. You want to cover all the dry ingredients with the nut butter mixture.

Transfer the mixture into the prepared loaf pan. Press evenly the mixture with your hand to leave no air. Flatten the surface with a spatula.

Freeze for 20 minutes until the breakfast bars are hard and set. Remove from the freezer, lift the parchment paper to pull out the bar from the loaf pan. Place on a plate. Sprinkle extra sliced almonds on top.

In a small bowl, microwave the sugar-free dark chocolate and coconut oil until fully melted.

Drizzle the melted chocolate on top of the bar, return into the freezer 1-3 minutes until the chocolate is set.

Cut into 8 breakfast bars.

Wrap each bar individually into plastic wrap or bee wax. Store in the fridge up to 8 days.

Nutrition Info

Calories 306 Calories from Fat 253 Fat 28.1g Carbohydrates 9.6g Fiber 6.8g Sugar 1.4g Protein 7.9g Net Carbs 2.8g

Vegan Black Bean Brownies

These easy Vegan Black Bean Brownies are a healthy chocolate dessert, low- calorie, low-carb and gluten-free with no added sugar, only 5 grams of net carbs per serve.

Prep Time: 10 mins Cook Time: 25 mins Total Time: 35 mins

Ingredients

Black Bean Brownies

1/4 cup Coconut oil + 1 teaspoon to grease pan

3.5 oz Sugar-free Dark Chocolate - see note for details 1 can Black beans , rinsed, drained (15 oz)

1 cup Almond Flour

3/4 cup Unsweetened apple sauce

1 teaspoon Baking Powder Caramelized Pecan

1 teasponn Coconut oil

1/4 cup peacan roughly chopped

2 tablespoon Sugar-free flavored maple syrup Dark Chocolate Drizzle

1 oz Sugar-free Dark Chocolate , melted, - see note for options

Black Bean Brownies

Instructions

Preheat oven to 300F (150C).

Line an 8 inches x 8 inches square brownie pan with parchment paper. Rub a little coconut oil on it to make sure it does not stick. Set aside.

In a small mixing bowl, add dark chocolate and coconut oil, microwave by 30-second bursts, stir and repeat until fully melted. If you don't have a microwave use a saucepan and melt under low heat until fully melted. Set aside.

In a food processor, with the S blade attachment, add all the ingredients: melted oil/chocolate mixture, black beans, baking powder, almond meal unsweetened applesauce

Pour into the prepared pan and spread evenly. Bake for 25-30 minutes max.

Cool down 5 minutes in the pan then lift out the parchment paper to unmold the brownie.

Place the brownie on a rack, drizzle extra melted chocolate on top if you like. I melted my chocolate in a small bowl in the microwave. Go with 30-second burst, stir, repeat until melted and drizzle over the brownie!

Caramelized Pecan Nuts

Melt coconut oil in a small frying pan over low heat.

Add roughly chopped pecan nuts and maple syrup.

Cook for 2 to 3 minutes, stirring constantly until it caramelizes. Spread out on parchment paper to cool.

Sprinkle over the brownie after drizzling the melted chocolate. This brownie is getting super fudgy when stored in the fridge. I recommend to store in an airtight plastic box in the fridge up to 3 days or in a cookie jar in the pantry.

Chocolate options: You can use any chocolate in this recipe. I tested 70% cocoa dark chocolate which gives the perfect sweetness, it's sugar-free and it gives a perfectly sweet brownie without the extra carbs or sugar (get Sugar Free Lillys Bars here affiliate link). You can also use 85% cocoa chocolate for a bitter/less sweet brownie.

Sugar free/low carb: don't use maple syrup to caramelize the nuts. Use same amount of sugar free crystal sweetener like swerve.

Nutrition Info

Fat 7.3g11% Carbohydrates 8.7g3% Fiber 3.5g15%

Sugar 1.3g1% Protein 3.2g6% Net Carbs 5.2g

Simple nutty pancakes

Prep: 5 mins Cook:5 mins easy makes 4 Ingredients

150g self-raising flour

½ tsp baking powder

1 large egg 150ml milk

2 tbsp agave syrup, plus extra to serve

50 g mixed nuts, chopped

2 tbsp rapeseed oil, for frying

Directions:

Tip the flour and baking powder into a large bowl with a pinch of salt. Make a well in the centre, then add the egg, milk and syrup. Whisk until smooth, then fold in half the nuts.

Heat 1 tbsp oil in a large, non-stick frying pan over a medium-high heat. Spoon two ladles of the mixture into the pan and cook for 1 min each side. Repeat to make two more.

Serve with a drizzle of agave syrup and the remaining nuts for extra crunch.

Flowerpot chocolate chip muffins

Prep: 10 mins Cook:12 mins - 15 mins Easy Makes 10 mini-muffins

Ingredients

3 tbsp vegetable oil

125g plain flour

1 tsp baking powder

25g cocoa powder

100g golden caster sugar

1 large egg 100ml milk 150g milk chocolate chips

25g chocolate cake decorations such as vermicelli sprinkles or chocolate-coated popping candy

20 rice paper wafer daisies (these come in packs of 12, so get 2 packs)

10 mini teracotta pots

Directions:

Heat oven to 180C/160C fan/gas 4. Lightly oil the inside of the terracotta pots with a little vegetable oil and place on a baking tray. Place a paper mini muffin case in the bottom of each pot.

Put the flour, baking powder and cocoa in a bowl and stir in the sugar.

Crack the egg into a jug and whisk with the milk and remaining oil. Pour this over the flour and cocoa mixture, and stir in with 50g of the chocolate chips. Be careful not to overmix – you want a loose but still quite lumpy mixture. Spoon into the pots up to three- quarters complete. Place in the middle of the oven and bake for 12-15 mins until risen and firm. Transfer to a wire rack (still in the pots) and leave to cool.

Put the rest of the chocolate chips in a small bowl and melt over a small pan of gently simmering water (don't let the water touch the bowl), or put in a microwave-proof bowl and heat on High for 1 min until melted.

Spread the tops of the muffins with the melted chocolate. Sprinkle over the chocolate decorations and add 2 rice paper wafer daisies to each pot to serve. Will keep for 2 days in an airtight container.

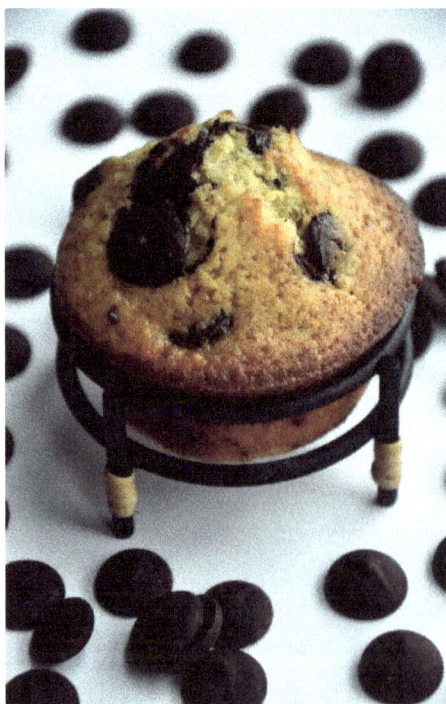

Sticky plum flapjack bars

Prep:20 mins Cook:1 hr Easy Makes 18

Ingredients

450g fresh plum, halved, stoned and roughly sliced

½ tsp mixed spice 300g light muscovado sugar

350g butter 300g rolled porridge oats (not jumbo)

140g plain flour 50g chopped walnut pieces

3 tbsp golden syrup

Directions:

Heat oven to 200C/180C fan/gas 6. Tip the plums into a bowl. Toss with the spice, 50g of the sugar and a small pinch of salt, then set aside to macerate.

Gently melt the butter in a saucepan. In a large bowl, mix the oats, flour, walnut pieces and remaining sugar, making sure there are no lumps of sugar, then stir in the butter and golden syrup until everything is combined into a loose flapjack mixture.

Grease a square baking tin about 20 x 20cm. Press half the oaty mix over the base of the tin, then tip over the plums and spread to make an even layer. Press the remaining oats over the plums so they are entirely covered right to the sides of the tin. Bake for 45-50 mins until dark golden and starting to crisp a little around the edges. Leave to cool completely, then cut into 18 little bars. Will keep in an airtight container for 2 days or can be frozen for up to a month.

Easter chocolate bark

Prep: 20 mins Cook:5 mins plus cooling easy Makes enough for 6-8 gift bags

Ingredients

3 x 200g bars milk chocolate

2 x 90g packs mini chocolate eggs

1 heaped tsp freeze-dried raspberry pieces – or you could use crystallised petals

Directions:

Break the chocolate into a large heatproof bowl. Bring a pan of water to a simmer, then sit the bowl on top. The water must not touch the bottom of the bowl. Let the chocolate slowly melt, stirring now and again with a spatula. For best results, temper your chocolate (see tip).

Meanwhile, lightly grease then line a 23 x 33cm roasting tin or baking tray with parchment. Put three-quarters of the mini eggs into a food bag and bash them with a rolling pin until broken up a little.

When the chocolate is smooth, pour it into the tin. Tip the tin from side to side to let the chocolate find the corners and level out. Scatter with the smashed and whole mini eggs, followed by the freeze- dried raspberry pieces. Leave to set, then remove from the parchment and snap into shards, ready to pack in boxes or bags.

Chocolate fudge cupcakes

Prep:30 mins Cook:25 mins - 30 mins easy Makes 12

Ingredients

200g butter 200g plain chocolate, under 70% cocoa solids is fin 200g light, soft brown sugar

2 eggs, beaten 1 tsp vanilla extract 250g self-raising flour

Smarties, sweets and sprinkles, to decorate

For the icing

200g plain chocolate 100ml double cream, not fridge-cold 50g icing sugar

Directions:

Heat oven to 160C/140C fan/gas 3 and line a 12-hole muffin tin with cases. Gently melt the butter, chocolate, sugar and 100ml hot water together in a large saucepan, stirring occasionally, then set aside to cool a little while you weigh the other ingredients.

Stir the eggs and vanilla into the chocolate mixture. Put the flour into a large mixing bowl, then stir in the chocolate mixture until smooth. Spoon into cases until just over three- quarters full, then set aside for 5 mins before putting on a low shelf in the oven and baking for 20-22 mins. Leave to cool.

For the icing, melt the chocolate in a heatproof bowl over a pan of barely simmering water. Once melted, turn off the heat, stir in the double cream and sift in the icing sugar. When spreadable, top each cake with some and decorate with your favourite sprinkles and sweets.

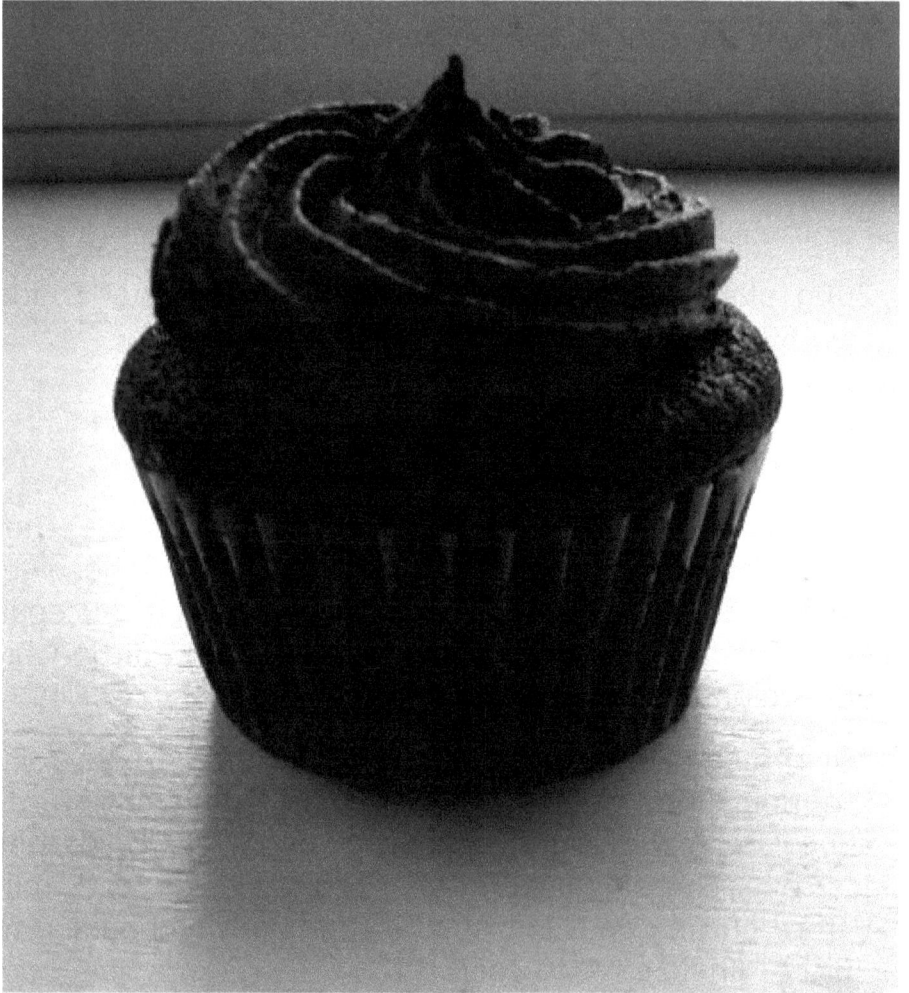

Dates and Almond Halwa

Prep time: 10 min Cooking Time: 20 min serve: 2

Ingredients

1 cup dates, dried, stemmed and coarsely chopped

½ cup water

½ cup almonds finely chopped

½ cup shelled pine nuts finely chopped

1 tablespoon coconut oil

¼ teaspoon cardamom ground

Instructions

Combine the dates and water in the Instant Pot.

Secure the lid and set the Pressure Release to Sealing. Select the Pressure Cook or Manual setting and set the cooking time for 5 minutes at High pressure.

Perform a quick release by moving the Pressure Release to Venting. Open the pot and coarsely mash the dates with a potato masher or wooden spatula.

Add the almonds, pine nuts, coconut oil, and cardamom and stir together.

Press the Cancel button to reset the cooking program, select the low Sauté setting and cook the Halwa, stirring frequently, until it thickens to a pudding-like consistency, about 10 minutes. Press the Cancel button to turn off the Instant Pot.

Spoon the Halwa into bowls and serve.

Nutrition Facts

Calories 339, Total Fat 7.2g, Saturated Fat 5.9g, Cholesterol 0mg , Sodium 4mg, Total Carbohydrate

66.8g, Dietary Fiber 7.1g, Total Sugars 56.4g, Protein 2.2g

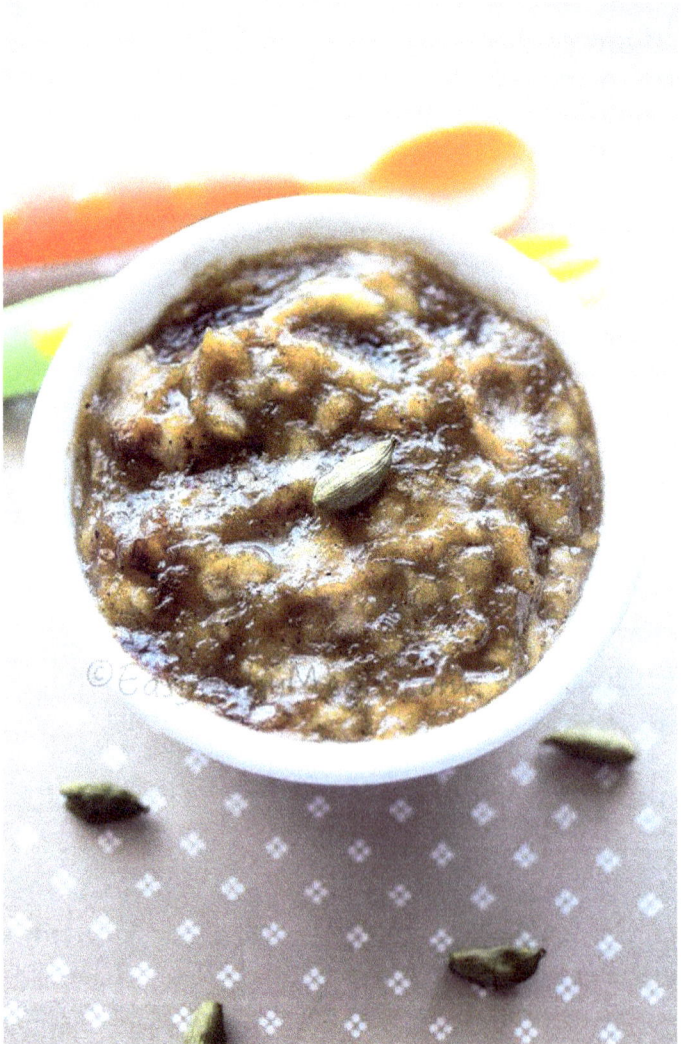

Fudge Pine nuts Brownies

Prep time: 10 min Cooking Time: 35 min serve: 2

Ingredients

½ cup oats flour

1/8 teaspoon baking powder

1/8 teaspoon salt

1 cup coconut sugar

½ cup coconut oil, softened

2 eggs

2 cups squares unsweetened baking chocolate, melted

½ teaspoon vanilla extract

1 cup coarsely chopped Pine nuts

1 cup water

Instructions

Grease an 8x8-inch square pan.

Sift oats flour, baking powder, and salt together in a bowl.

Beat coconut sugar and coconut oil together in a large bowl with an electric mixer until light and fluffy. Beat in eggs until smooth batter forms; beat in chocolate and vanilla extract. Stir oats flour mixture in just until incorporated; fold in pine nuts. Spread batter into prepared square pan.

Pour 1 cup water into the Instant Pot and arrange the handled trivet on the bottom. Place the pan on top of the trivet and cover it with an upside-down plate or another piece of parchment to protect the brownies from condensation.

Secure the lid and move the steam release valve to Sealing. Select Manual/Pressure Cook to cook on high pressure for 30 minutes. When the cooking cycle is complete, let the pressure naturally release for 10 minutes, then move the steam release valve to Venting to release any remaining pressure. When the floating valve drops, remove the lid.

Let the brownies cool completely in the pan before cutting and serving.

Nutrition Facts

Calories 346, Total Fat 29.5g, Saturated Fat 12.6g, Cholesterol 63mg, Sodium 134mg, Total Carbohydrate 14.5g, Dietary Fiber 0.6g , Total Sugars 12.9g, Protein 4.7g

Gooey brownies

Prep:10 mins Cook:35 mins easy Makes 16-20
Ingredients

100g unsalted butter, softened

175g caster sugar

2 large eggs, beaten

75g plain flour

50g cocoa powder

1 tsp baking powder

3 tbsp milk 4 tbsp mixed white and milk chocolate chips

100g milk chocolate 75g full-fat soft cheese

Directions:

Heat oven to 180C/160C fan/gas 4 and line a 20cm square brownie tin with baking parchment. Beat the butter and sugar together with an electric whisk, then add the eggs one by one.

Sift in the flour, cocoa powder and baking powder, and add the milk. Mix everything, then stir in the chocolate chips. Spoon into the tin and level the top. Bake for 30 mins, or until the top is set, then cool completely.

Meanwhile, make the topping, melt the milk chocolate, cool a little, then mix it with the soft cheese until thoroughly combined and silky.Spread the topping over the cooleed brownies and cut into small squares – these are very rich.

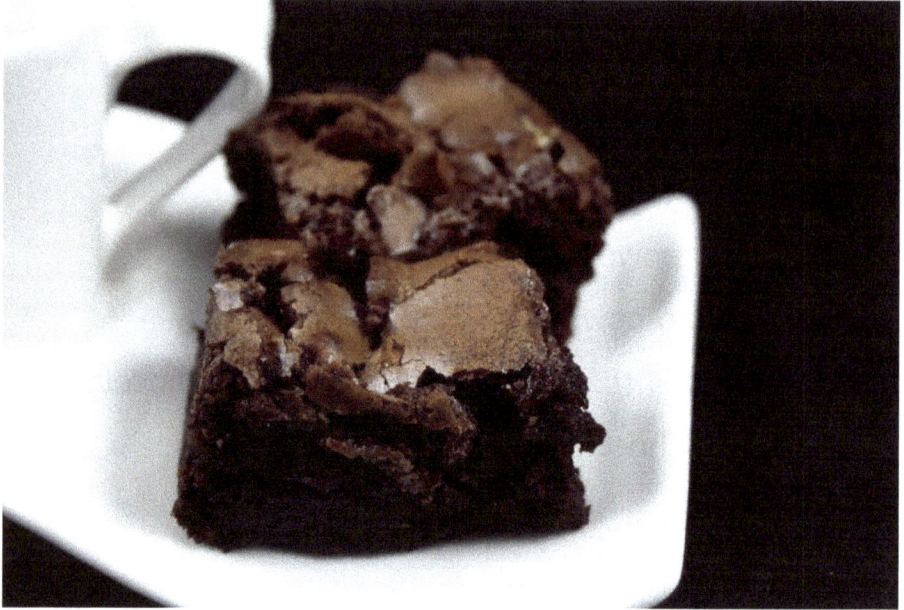

Mango crunch cookies

Prep: 15 mins Cook:15 mins plus chilling and cooling Easy Makes about 14 large or 28 small cookies

Ingredients

140g butter, at room temperature

50g golden caster sugar

1 egg yolk

1 tsp vanilla extract

1 tbsp maple syrup

100g dried mango, roughly chopped

175g plain flour, plus extra for dusting

To decorate (optional)

200g icing sugar, sifted

3 tbsp mango juice

sprinkles

Directions:

Heat the oven to 180C/160C fan/gas

Place the butter and sugar in a food processor and blitz until smooth and creamy.

Add the egg yolk, vanilla, maple syrup and mango. Whizz to blend in and chop the mango a little more finely. Add the flour and briefly blitz to form a soft dough. Turn out onto a floured surface and shape into a ball. Chill for 20 mins.Using a rolling pin, roll the cookie dough to the thickness of a £1 coin on a lightly floured surface, then cut out biscuit shapes with a 10cm cutter for large, or a 5cm cutter smaller cookies.

Transfer to a baking tray lined with baking parchment, and cook for 12-15 mins or until lightly golden and firm. Remove and leave to cool on a wire rack.

If decorating, mix the icing sugar with the mango juice to make a runny icing. Drizzle or spoon the icing over the biscuits, add the sprinkles if using, and leave to set. Will keep in a biscuit tin for up to 1 week.

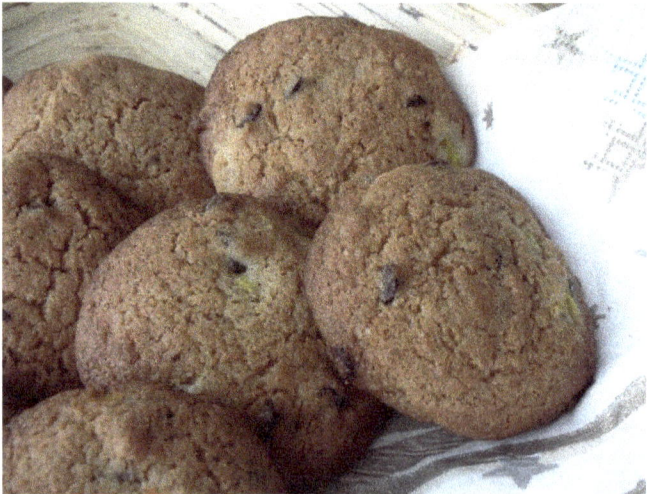

www.ingramcontent.com/pod-product-compliance
Lightning Source LLC
Chambersburg PA
CBHW050754030426
42336CB00012B/1811